MW01601733

Lifestyle Medicine for Chronic Diseases

Thomas L. Lenz

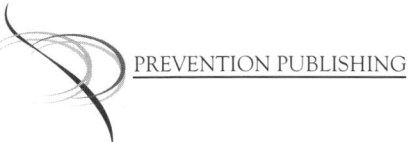

PREVENTION PUBLISHING

Omaha, Nebraska USA

Lifestyle Medicine for Chronic Diseases
By Thomas L. Lenz

Copyright © 2013 Prevention Publishing, Inc.

3606 North 156th Street
Suite 101-314
Omaha, NE 68116

Library of Congress Control Number: 2013905937
ISBN: 978-0-9825044-6-8

Printed in the United States of America

Disclaimer

The author, reviewers, and publisher are not responsible for errors or omissions or for consequences from application of the information in this book and make no warranty, expressed or implied, with respect to the currency, completeness, or accuracy of the contents of the publication. Application of the information in a particular situation remains the responsibility of the individual and his/her healthcare provider. The author and Prevention Publishing, Inc. disclaim all liability in connection with the use of the information in this book.

Cover design by Phil Beagle

To purchase additional copies, please visit
http://preventionpublishing.com

*This book is dedicated to my wife Nancy
and our four children Kaelie, Abbey, Jack, and Luke*

Preface

The Centers for Disease Control and Prevention (CDC) has stated that 7 out of 10 deaths and 75% of the total health care costs in the United States are due to chronic diseases. Nearly 1 out of every 2 Americans has at least one chronic disease. Almost 90% of heart attacks and strokes are due to preventable causes. The CDC has the following statement posted on their *Chronic Disease Prevention and Health Promotion* website: "Four modifiable health risk behaviors—lack of physical activity, poor nutrition, tobacco use, and excessive alcohol consumption—are responsible for much of the illness, suffering, and early death related to chronic diseases."[1]

Lifestyle medicine focuses on treating the true causes of chronic disease. Lifestyle medicine may be one of the only disease prevention and treatment modalities that crosscuts every health care profession and, if fully developed, has the potential to be the gold standard in interprofessional patient care. *Lifestyle Medicine for Chronic Diseases* was written for health care professionals to fill a void in the current formal and informal education of comprehensive lifestyle medicine practice. It can be used as a textbook with students in undergraduate, graduate or health professions programs. It can also be used and for professional development in those who have already completed their formal training, as well as for personal use to improve ones own health.

1. Centers for Disease Control and Prevention. Chronic Disease Prevention and Health Promotion. Available at: http://www.cdc.gov/chronicdisease/index.htm. Accessed on March 28, 2013.

Reviewers

Nicole D. White, PharmD
Omaha, Nebraska

Jessica C. Larson, PharmD
Marrero, Louisiana

Nancy J. Lenz, MA, MPT
Omaha, Nebraska

Contents

Section I

Overview of Lifestyle Medicine

1　Introduction to Lifestyle Medicine

> **Objectives**
> 1. Define lifestyle medicine.
> 2. Explain the impact of chronic diseases on the health care system in the United States.
> 3. Justify the use of lifestyle medicine to treat certain chronic diseases.

Lifestyle Medicine is defined by the American College of Lifestyle Medicine as, "the use of lifestyle interventions in the treatment and management of disease."[1] Lifestyle interventions can include activities such as healthy eating, exercise or physical activity, stress management, restorative sleep, tobacco cessation, alcohol moderation and a variety of other non-drug activities.[1] The essence of lifestyle medicine, from a health care professional's perspective, is the concept of preventing and treating the true "cause" of disease, rather than simply managing the symptoms of disease.

In 2007, two sociologists from Australia published a book entitled, *Lifestyle In Medicine*.[2] In their book, Hansen and Easthope present the idea that preventing and treating disease using lifestyle activities focuses on the future, and the advancement of health. They provide the following explanation:

> *"...because lifestyle models provide an explanation for poor health where the factors considered to be determinants of disease are commonly perceived to be modifiable, a lifestyle approach is often oriented towards the future and emphasizes the maintenance and fostering of health."[2]*

What Hansen and Easthope are saying is that lifestyle medicine is a fundamental change in our thinking about disease as health care professionals. When we use lifestyle medicine to prevent and treat disease, our focus is on what is yet to come rather than what has already happened. For example, with lifestyle medicine we think about heart disease differently - our focus is on preventing a heart attack, rather than reacting to one after it has occurred. Our current health care system (and the education system that trains its professionals) focuses on providing the best care possible to patients who have had a heart attack. Focusing on the future is one of the fundamental tenants of lifestyle medicine. This changes the mindset of our health care and education systems to train health care professionals to prevent the heart attack from occurring in the first place.

Another way to look at this is to visualize a long distance running event, such as a marathon. The current leaders of the race are cardiovascular disease, cancer, stroke, obesity, diabetes and many other chronic diseases. Our current health care system is also in the race, but is desperately trying to catch up with the leaders. To no avail, our current system continues to fall further behind the leaders because its race strategy is to react to adverse heath events (e.g. heart attack) after they happen. A more effective race strategy may be to initiate health care practices that affect the true "causes" of disease, thereby preventing or significantly delaying them from occurring. If lifestyle medicine was at the core of our health care system, it would take the lead in the race. Strategies that emphasize prevention are oriented towards the future, rather than reacting to the past.

A second major tenant of lifestyle medicine is also mentioned by Hansen and Easthope when they talk about "...the maintenance and fostering of health." Lifestyle medicine encourages the advancement of health, not just the treatment of illness. Our current health care system is often referred to as a "sick care" system rather than a "health care" system. Incorporating lifestyle medicine into mainstream health care practices changes our focus to one that strives for optimal health not just the absence of disease. As we will discuss later, optimal health is different for each individual. Optimizing lifestyle medicine activities improves quality of life at all ages and all stages of life. Lifestyle medicine cultivates, strengthens and enriches a healthy life.

4

State of Our Health

In 2005, chronic diseases affected about 133 million Americans, or about 45% of the population.[3,4] The prevalence of chronic disease increases with age. Approximately 25% of young adults have one or more chronic disease(s). This increases to 50% in middle-aged adults and to 69% in elderly adults in the United States.[3,4] In 2005, nearly 1 out of every 2 American adults had at least one chronic disease.[3] Moreover, about 1 in 4 Americans with a chronic disease say that their daily activities are negatively effected by their condition.

> ✓**Fast Fact:** 75% of the total health care costs in the U.S. are related to preventable conditions.[3]

The financial burden on the health care system as a result of chronic diseases is significant. In 2004, chronic diseases accounted for $1.7 trillion in health case expenditures, or about 75% of all health care costs in the United States.[4] At an individual level, this amounted to about $6,280 per person per year.[4]

In 2009, chronic diseases accounted for 70% of all deaths. In fact, during that same year, 4 out of 5 deaths was a chronic disease.[4] The most recent data shows that the top 5 causes of death are:

> #1 Heart Disease
> #2 Cancer
> #3 Stroke
> #4 Chronic Respiratory Disease
> #5 Unintentional Injury

Additionally, a study published in 2009 concluded that only 7.5% of American adults were considered to have a low-risk factor burden for heart disease.[5] This means that only 7.5% of Americans meet all 5 of the following criteria: at recommended levels (or not taking medications) for high blood cholesterol and high blood pressure, a body mass index indicating no overweight or obesity, not currently smoking, and not having previously been diagnosed with diabetes.[5]

> **√ *Fast Fact:*** Only 5.1% of American adults without cardiovascular disease do not smoke AND get the recommended amounts of physical activity, fruits and vegetables simultaneously.[6]

Drug Therapy and Health Care

As already proposed, our current health care system has been re-actionary to disease and focuses on treating illnesses once they occur. Over the past several decades there has been a great deal of focus on drug development for the treatment of acute and chronic diseases. There is no doubt that advancements in drug therapy have lead to a more effective management of almost every disease. But, drug development comes at a high price.

The 2012 Pharmaceutical Industry Profile from the Pharmaceutical Research and Manufacturers of America (PhRMA) reports that it takes 10 to 15 years and costs $1.2 billion to fully develop and prepare one innovative new drug for the marketplace.[7] In 2011, members of PhRMA spent $49.5 billion on research and development. The number of new drugs in development in 2012 for several common chronic diseases is as follows:

•Cancer: 948
•Respiratory Disorders: 398
•Mental Disorders: 255
•Cardiovascular Disorders: 252
•HIV/AIDS: 88
•Arthritis: 76
•Alzheimer's Disease: 72

The drug industry is vital to our health care system. However, it provides us with a good example of how our system is set up to be a disease reactionary system - and it's expensive. Perhaps, this should lead us to the conclusion that there may be a better way forward for our health care system. Increasing our efforts to prevent disease may help us win the race against chronic disease and prove to be more cost effective as a result.

> ✓ *Fast Fact:* The U.S. only spends 3% of its total health care dollars on disease prevention efforts.[3]

Forecasting the Future of Health in America

Cardiovascular disease (CVD) encompasses a group of disorders that involve the heart and blood vessels. Although various organizations define CVD differently, it generally includes the conditions of hypertension, coronary heart disease (CHD), heart failure, stroke, peripheral vascular disease and others. Diseases related to the heart have been listed as the most common cause of death among Americans since the early 1900s when it took over the top spot from infectious disease related illnesses. In 2010, the American Heart Association (AHA) reported that 36.9% of Americans had CVD and predicted that by 2030, 40.5% of the U.S. population will have some form of CVD.[8] Specifically, hypertension, CHD, heart failure and stroke are expected to increase by 9.9%, 16.6%, 25%, and 24.9%, respectively.[8] This translates to an extra 27 million Americans with hypertension in 2030 compared with 2010. The same can be said for an extra 8 million with CHD, 4 million with stroke and 3 million with heart failure.[8]

Additionally, between 2010 and 2030, the total annual direct medical costs associated with CVD are projected to triple from $273 billion to $818 billion. Indirect costs (due to lost productivity) associated with CVD are expected to increase by over 60% from $172 billion in 2010 to $276 billion in 2030.[8] Because of its higher prevalence, hypertension is the most expensive component of CVD.[8]

Diabetes is also quickly becoming a significant health concern due to the debilitating nature of the disease and its increasing prevalence. It is currently the 7th leading cause of death in America and about 1 in 10 adults have a diagnosis of diabetes.[9] People with diabetes have medical costs that are more than twice that of people without diabetes. The Centers for Disease Control and Prevention (CDC) predicts that by the year 2050, as many as 1 in 3 American adults will have diabetes.[9] The International Diabetes Federation predicts that diabetes will increase by 54% worldwide by the year 2030.[9]

Making the Case for Lifestyle Medicine

Diseases related to the heart have been the most common cause of death over the past century. However, if we are to place a greater emphasis on disease prevention, we need to look closer at the "actual" reasons why people die from heart disease and other conditions. In 2005, the CDC published results from an analysis that compared the "leading" causes of death to the "actual" causes of death in the U.S.[10,11] The results of their analysis showed the following:

Leading Causes of Death
#1 Heart disease
#2 Cancer
#3 Stroke
#4 Chronic respiratory disease
#5 Unintentional injury

Actual Causes of Death
#1 Tobacco use
#2 Poor diet and physical inactivity
#3 Alcohol consumption
#4 Microbial agents
#5 Toxic agents

In looking at this comparison, we can easily see that although the leading causes of death are CVD and cancer-related, the "actual" reasons for death appear to be related to lifestyle behaviors. If we want to look even closer at this issue, we should try to answer the questions of why people are using tobacco, eating poorly, being physically inactive and consuming too much alcohol.

In 2004, *The Lancet* published the INTERHEART study which aimed to determine the strength of association between various risk factors and acute myocardial infarction (heart attack).[12] In 2010, *The Lancet* published a similar analysis for stroke called the INTER-STROKE study.[13] Both of these studies found that 90% or more of heart attacks and strokes can be attributed to 10 modifiable risk factors. These risk factors include abnormal blood lipids (cholesterol), smoking, hypertension, diabetes, abdominal obesity, psychosocial factors (e.g. stress and depression), low consumption of fruits and vegetables, over consumption of alcohol, and a lack of physical activity.[12,13] Most of these are lifestyle related behaviors and the chronic diseases identified on the list can be significantly modified with positive lifestyle behaviors.

Evidence-based medicine is a concept in patient care where a health care professional uses scientific evidence to make clinical decisions. All health care providers are encouraged by their respective professions to practice evidence-based medicine. Practice guideline recommendations are published by various organizations such as the National Institutes of Health, Heart, Lung and Blood Institute and the American Diabetes Association to guide health care professionals in practicing evidence-based medicine. An overall review of the practice guidelines for several chronic diseases shows that nearly all guidelines recommend lifestyle medicine related behaviors to both prevent and treat disease.[14]

The following is a list of chronic diseases in which the clinical guidelines, from their respective organizations, recommend lifestyle modifications for BOTH prevention and treatment of the condition:

- Hypertension
- Dyslipidemia
- Heart Disease
- Stroke
- Peripheral Arterial Disease
- Heart Failure
- Diabetes Type 2
- Obesity
- Metabolic Syndrome
- Osteoporosis
- Osteoarthritis

Lastly, a study published in 2011 looked at the combined effect of four lifestyle medicine related behaviors to all-cause mortality (death from any cause).[15] The four lifestyle medicine related behaviors included never having smoked, maintaining a healthy diet, getting adequate physical activity, and consuming no more than moderate amounts of alcohol. The results showed people who practiced all four behaviors were 63% less likely to die of any cause, compared with people who did not participate in any of the four behaviors. Additionally, those who did not participate in any of the four lifestyle medicine behaviors had an increased risk of dying equal to over 11 years of chronological age compared with those who participated in all four.[15] This study demonstrates that participating in multiple lifestyle behaviors can have a powerful affect on mortality.

Summary Points

- Lifestyle medicine involves several non-drug activities that aim to treat the true cause of disease.
- Lifestyle medicine focuses on the advancement of the future health of an individual.
- Chronic diseases are a significant burden at an individual level and to the U.S. health care system.
- Few Americans are considered to have low-risk for CHD and few participate in lifestyle medicine activities.
- A great deal of money is spent by our health care system to be reactive to disease, rather than proactive and preventive.
- By 2030, over 40% of U.S. adults may have CVD and by 2050, over 30% of Americans may have diabetes.
- The actual causes of death are due to a lack of lifestyle medicine related activities.
- Evidence-based practice guidelines recommend lifestyle medicine activities for the prevention and treatment of disease.

Test Your Knowledge

---

1. The overall percentage of the American population who are affected by at least one chronic disease is:

a. 10%
b. 25%
© 45%
d. 65%

2. According to the CDC, the #1 actual cause of death is:

a. Tobacco use
b. Microbial agents
c. Toxic agents
d. Motor vehicle accidents

3. Studies have shown that _____% or more of heart attacks and strokes can be attributed to _____ modifiable risk factors.

a. 50%, 5
b. 40%, 7
c. 60%, 3
d. 90%, 10

Practical Application Tools

Lifestyle Journal. Using a log book or journal can be an effective method to keep track of a variety of healthy lifestyle related activities, such as nutrition. A comprehensive journal that incorporates several lifestyle medicine related activities can be an effective tool for the patient to improve lifestyle habit self-awareness and lifestyle medicine program adherence. A lifestyle journal can also be an effective tool from the health care provider's perspective as a means to keep track of patient self-reported behaviors and patient accountability to a lifestyle medicine program. An example of a lifestyle journal is provided in Toolbox A.

Composite Lifestyle Index. Many people think of healthy lifestyle activities as only proper nutrition and exercise. While these components are important, other activities such as stress management, sleep success, alcohol moderation and tobacco abstinence are also important to maintaining a healthy lifestyle. It doesn't make sense to concentrate on only one or two of these components and ignore the rest. If we achieve an acceptable level of success with several (or all) of these activities, overall health could be greater than if a high level of just one activity is achieved. The Composite Lifestyle Index (CLI) was developed as a scoring tool to help quantify a balanced healthy lifestyle. Six CLI components (physical activity, healthy eating, sleep, stress, alcohol consumption, and tobacco use) are used to measure overall balance. Each of the six components is scored on a scale from 0-10 or 1-10 and is based on an individuals participation in the activities over the previous two weeks. A possible total score of 60 can be achieved, and the objective is to get the highest score possible. A score of 20 points should be an initial goal with a score of 40 points or more, being the ultimate goal. The CLI is unique because it provides a single number that represents comprehensive lifestyle medicine participation - similar to how a student's grade point average represents comprehensive academic performance. Initial research on the CLI shows that a higher score is related to a greater overall health related quality of life.[16] The CLI scoring tables are provided in Toolbox B.

References

1. American College of Lifestyle Medicine. What is Lifestyle Medicine? Available at: http://www.lifestylemedicine.org/define. Accessed on: November 30, 2012.
2. Hansen E, Easthope G. Lifestyle In Medicine. Routledge. Oxon, New York. 2007.
3. Centers for Disease Control and Prevention. Chronic Disease Prevention and Health Promotion. Available at: http://www.cdc.gov/chronicdisease/index.htm. Accessed on: November 30, 2012.
4. Partnership to Fight Chronic Disease. 2009 Almanac of Chronic Disease. Available at: http://www.fightchronicdisease.org/ resources/ almanac -chronic-disease-0. Accessed on: November 30, 2012.
5. Ford ES, Li C, Zhao G, Pearson WS, Capewell S. Trends in the prevalence of low risk factor burden for cardiovascular disease among United States adults. Circulation. 2009;120:1181-1188.
6. Miller RR, Sales AE, Kopjar B, Fihn SD, Bryson CL. Adherence to heart-healthy behaviors in a sample of the U.S. population. Prev Chronic Dis 2005 April. Available at: URL: http://www.cdc.gov/ pcd/issues/2005/apr/04_0115.htm. Accessed on: December 2, 2012.
7. Pharmaceutical Research and Manufactures of America. PhRMA 2012 Pharmaceutical Industry Profile. Available at: http://phrma.org. Accessed on: December 2, 2012.
8. Heidenreich PA, Trogdon JG, Khavjou OA, Butler J, Dracup K, et al. Forecasting the future of cardiovascular disease in the United States. A

policy statement from the American Heart Association. Circulation. 2011;123:933-944.

9. Boyle JP, Thompson TJ, Gregg EW, Baker LE, Williamson DF. Projection of the year 2050 burden of diabetes in the US adult population: dynamic modeling of incidence, mortality, and prediabetes prevalence. Population Health Matrics. 2010;8:29.

10. Mokdad AH, Marks JS, Stroup DF, Gerberding JL. Actual causes of death in the United States, 2000. JAMA. 2004;291:1238-1246.

11. Mokdad AH. Correction: Actual causes of death in the United States, 2000. JAMA. 2005;293:298.

12. Yusef S, Hawken S, Oupuu S, Dans T, et al. Effect of potentially modifiable risk factors associated with myocardial infarction in 52 countries (the INTERHEART study): case-control study. Lancet. 2004;364:937-952.

13. Tu JV. Reducing global burden of stroke: INTERSTROKE. Lancet. 2010; published online June 18, 2010. DOI:10.1016/ S0140-6736(10)60834-3.

14. Lenz TL, Petersen K, Monaghan MS. Counseling patients about lifestyle modification. US Pharmacist. 2008;33(1):38-45.

15. Ford ES, Zhao G, Tsai J, Li C. Low-risk lifestyle behaviors and all cause mortality: Findings from the National Health and Nutrition Examination Survey III Mortality Study. Am J Public Health. 2011;101(10):1922-1929.

16. Lenz TL, Gillespie ND, Skradski JJ, Viereck LK, Packard KA, Monaghan MS. Development of a composite lifestyle index and its relationship to quality of life improvement: The CLI pilot study. ISRN Preventive Medicine. 2013;volume 2013:Article ID 481030.

Section II

Core Elements of Lifestyle Medicine

2 Health Behavior Modification

Objectives

1. Explain the concept of self-efficacy and its importance to behavior change theories.
2. Describe the stages of the Transtheoretical Model of Behavior Change.
3. Describe the importance of identifying individually specific behavior change barriers.

Health behavior modification may be the single most important fundamental concept in lifestyle medicine. If it is true that 75% of our total health care costs are related to preventable conditions (presented in the previous chapter), then it is logical to assume that a conscious decision or behavior is the primary cause of the preventable condition. Therefore, understanding why people make the choices they do regarding their health, becomes important for us as health care providers. Simply telling a patient that exercise is a good thing, and therefore should be done on a daily basis, is not necessarily quality patient care. Yet, this is the extent of the advice many patients receive from their health care providers.

A few years ago, my colleague and I conducted a study to assess the kind of advice patients who were newly diagnosed with hypercholesterolemia were getting regarding ways to lower their cholesterol, other than taking their medications.[1] We were encouraged to find that almost 3 out of 4 patients were receiving information regarding lifestyle modifications. However, for the majority of these patients, the total time spent discussing these strategies with their health care provider was less than 10 minutes in length.[1] Furthermore, only one-half of the patients who originally received lifestyle medicine-related information, received follow-up information from their health care provider. A significant number of patients received their follow-up lifestyle medicine related information from internet websites.[1]

It is not enough for health care providers to simply tell their patients that they need to stop smoking, exercise and eat better. We need to help them through this process with the understanding that it may take many years, even a lifetime, to consistently implement healthy lifestyle behaviors. A first rate exercise and nutrition prescription is all for not if we do not provide the patient with the knowledge, awareness and skills to be successful with the program. The purpose of this chapter is to provide information and tools that health care professionals can use with their patients to optimize lifestyle medicine program outcomes.

Adherence

The World Health Organization (WHO) defines adherence as the "extent to which a person's behavior - taking medication, following a diet, and/or executing lifestyle changes - corresponds with agreed recommendations from a health care provider."[2] The term adherence may be a better term to use than compliance, as adherence implies active participation while compliance implies a passive role. From a patient's perspective, it may make sense for us to use the term "adherence" because the word can mean "to stick to" or "to adhere to." Sticking to a lifestyle medicine program should be a message we are sending to our patients.

Although taking medications is not necessarily a lifestyle behavior, it is a behavior that requires adherence. Much data exists in the literature regarding medication adherence. Knowing how adults adhere to taking their medications, can help us better understand adherence related to lifestyle medicine behaviors. It is estimated that only 50% of patients with chronic conditions are adherent to taking their medications as prescribed.[3]

✓ **Fast Fact:** Medication non-adherence costs an estimated $100 billion per year in hospital admissions.[4]

One can argue that it may be easier to take a medication than participate in a healthy lifestyle behavior, such as eating more vegetables. If this is true, adherence rates to lifestyle medicine activities may be lower than medication adherence rates. It is reported that 79% of Americans adhere to the recommendation not to smoke.[5] In addition, almost 21% adhere to the recommendations for physical activity and 23.5% to fruit and vegetable consumption recommendations.[5] As discussed in Chapter 1, smoking, poor diet and physical inactivity are the most common "actual" causes of death in America.[6] Therefore, simultaneous adherence to all three of these activities is important. The Behavior Risk Factor Surveillance System (BRFSS) reports that only 5.1% of Americans without coronary heart disease adhere to all three activities at the same time.[7] The adherence rate for those with coronary heart disease is slightly higher at 7.2%.[7] This data shows that overall adherence rates to lifestyle medicine activities are low. Therefore, an understanding of health behavior modifications is an important topic for health care providers to maximize patient adherence to lifestyle medicine related behaviors.

Health Behavior Modification Theories

Several theories have been developed that attempt to explain the complex process of behavior modification. We are primarily interested in the theories that are health related, and in particular those that have been used in disease-prevention models. Two behavior change theories that are particularly applicable to lifestyle medicine are the Social Cognitive Theory and the Transtheoretical Model of Behavior Change.

Social Cognitive Theory

The Social Cognitive Theory is applicable for lifestyle medicine because it provides a framework for what is at the heart of lifestyle behavior change - the understanding, predicting and changing of human behavior.[8] As already mentioned, health care providers may not be providing the best care by simply telling a patient that they need to get more exercise. Quality, patient-centered care involves providing patients with the tools they need to be successful with an exercise program and other lifestyle medicine activities. Knowing why the individual is sedentary in the first place, and which behavior change strategies may work best, becomes very important for program success. Fundamental to the Social Cognitive Theory is the notion that human behavior is dependent upon one's own personal values, one's behaviors and experiences, and one's environment.[8] Human behavior, or behavior change, is based upon observing the behavior of others, the potential for self-directed changes in behavior, and through a process of self-reflection.[8]

The principle of self-efficacy is critical to the concept of the Social Cognitive Theory.[8] Self-efficacy, in itself, is a theory that states that for an individual to make a change, that individual must believe in themselves and have confidence that they can execute the desired behavior.[8] For self-efficacy, the individual (i.e. patient) is at the center of the behavior change process.[8] In adopting the principles of the Social Cognitive Theory for lifestyle medicine behavior change, the patient is at the center of the behaviors. The health care provider acts as a facilitator to lifestyle medicine activities by providing the necessary education, support and tools to the patient to help them make the decision to exercise, for example. The patient is then taught to be aware of their actions, their surroundings and to reflect on experiences in a way that can help them make an initial decision to exercise and to maintain an exercise program. Specific lifestyle medicine tools that may work well to apply this theory include self-monitoring journals, logbooks and self-reflection techniques. As the patient begins to understand why they make the decisions they do, they can become more self-aware, self-confident, and therefore, self-efficacious.

Transtheoretical Model of Behavior Change

The Transtheoretical Model (TTM) describes the stages that an individual goes through on their way towards implementing a new behavior, such as quitting tobacco use.[9] The Transtheoretical Model regards change not as a single event or moment, but rather a process that unfolds over time. Ideally, behavior change involves continual forward progress. Occasionally, however, previous unhealthy habits are resumed as a coping mechanism to manage stress, boredom, loneliness, anger, or depression. There are six "stages of readiness to change" in TTM and they are:[9]

1. Precontemplation. The patient is not intending to take action on a particular behavior within at least the next 6 months. Patients may be in this stage due to lack of education or because they feel demoralized from previous behavior change failures. They tend to avoid talking, thinking or reading about particular behaviors and are often classified as "resistant" and "unmotivated."

2. Contemplation. The patient is intending to make a change in the next 6 months. The individual is more aware of the positive aspects of the behavior change, but is also acutely aware of the negative aspects. Many patients can be stuck in this stage for a long time due to indecisiveness.

3. Preparation. The patient is intending to make a change in the next month and has a plan of action. The plan can include joining a gym, talking to a health care professional, buying a self-help book, and many others.

4. Action. The patient has made a specific behavior modification within the previous 6 months. The behavior change must meet criteria that scientists and professionals agree is sufficient to reduce health risk.

5. Maintenance. The patient is increasingly more confident that he/she can continue his/her behavior change and has consistently participated in the behavior for at least 6 months. It is estimated that this stage lasts from 6 months to 5 years.

6. Termination. Patients in this stage have zero temptation to discontinue the behavior change and have100% self-efficacy. Previous unhealthy habits are NOT resumed as a coping mechanism to manage stress, boredom, loneliness, anger, or depression.

One of the keys to using TTM in practice is to first assess an individual's TTM stage in one or more behaviors.[9] When discussing this with patients, it may be better to phrase your assessment as their "readiness to participate" rather than "readiness to change." (many people react negatively when they think someone is trying to "change" them, even if they volunteer to participate in a lifestyle medicine behavior change program) This assessment can then be coupled with their "confidence to participate" in one or more behaviors. Toolbox C provides examples of "Readiness to Participate" and "Confidence to Participate" questionnaires.

✓ **Fast Fact:** Approximately 40% of current smokers in America are in the precontemplation stage, 40% in the contemplation stage, and only 20% in the preparation stage.[9]

Barriers to Health Behavior Modification

An important personalized lifestyle medicine strategy that can be employed by health care professionals is to help patients identify and overcome their individual barriers to lifestyle medicine implementation and adherence. Barriers are inherent to any kind of behavior modification and no individual is immune to barriers. Some barriers can be simple and easy to resolve, while others are more complex and take time to overcome. Key to the process, however, is the ability to identify and develop solutions to patient specific barriers. Working one-on-one with a patient regarding this aspect of health behavior modification can truly make the difference between program adherence and non-adherence.

Health Coach

Health coaching, also called wellness coaching, is quickly becoming a popular component of lifestyle medicine. A health coach specializes in helping patients (or clients) achieve healthy lifestyle behaviors through techniques such as motivational interviewing, positive psychology and goal setting. Health coaching is not the same as psychotherapy or social work. A health coach's goal is to maximize patient self-efficacy towards positive health behaviors through a long-term coaching-type relationship. Many groups have incorporated health coaching into their chronic disease programs. Certifications are currently available in health and wellness coaching.

Summary Points

●Health behavior modification may be the most important concept in lifestyle medicine.
●Only 50% of patients with chronic conditions are adherent to their prescribed medications.
● Only 5.1% of Americans without CHD are simultaneously adherent to the recommended amounts of physical activity, fruit and vegetable consumption and do not smoke.

•Self-efficacy is an important behavior change concept and states that an individual must believe in himself/herself and have confidence that he/she can execute the desired behavior to be successful.

•The Social Cognitive Theory of behavior change fits well with lifestyle medicine activities because it suggests that the more the patient understands about himself/herself, the more likely he/she is to make positive lifestyle choices.

•The Transtheoretical Model of behavior change identifies six stages that a person will go through on their way to implementing and adhering to a new behavior.

•It is important to help patients identify and develop solutions to their specific lifestyle medicine activity barriers.

Test Your Knowledge

1. The percentage of Americans without CHD who adhere to the recommendations of all 3 health behaviors of smoking cessation, physical activity, and adequate fruit and vegetable intake is:

a. 50.4%
b. 25.3%
c. 10.7%
d. 5.1%

2. All of the following are stages of The Transtheoretical Model EXCEPT:

a. Pre-contemplation
b. Contemplation
c. Pre-preparation
d. Preparation
e. Action

3. The concept of self-efficacy can only be used in the Social Cognitive Theory of behavior change.

a. True
b. False

- criticle in Social Cognitive Theory of behavior Δ, but can be used in both

Practical Application Tools

Readiness and Confidence to Participate in Healthy Lifestyle Behaviors. The Transtheoretical Model (TTM) of behavior change presents six stages that people go through on their journey towards the implementation and adherence of a new behavior.[9] This process can take many years, perhaps even a lifetime. One of the advantages of TTM is that it provides a description (including a timeframe) of each stage that can be understood in practical terms at the patient level. Because of this, health care professionals can design a questionnaire specific to their program that allows their patients to "stage" their own readiness and confidence to participate in specific behaviors. Toolbox C provides an example of a *Readiness to Participate in Healthy Lifestyle Behaviors* questionnaire and a *Confidence to Participate in Healthy Lifestyle Behaviors* questionnaire.

The two questionnaires can be used in tandem when working with patients. The questionnaires should first be designed to fit the specific needs of a program by listing pertinent lifestyle medicine behaviors. The questionnaires can be administered when initiating a patient to a new program and at periodic time points - such as every 6 months. The results obtained from the questionnaires can be used to help choose the lifestyle medicine activities to implement first as well as a tool to track the progress of the patient's behavior change over time.

First, have the patient complete the *Readiness* questionnaire followed by the *Confidence* questionnaire. Next, look at the rankings in the *Readiness* questionnaire and make note of the activities that are ranked as a "4," "5" or "6." These are the lifestyle medicine activities that the patient is already doing. Compare these activities with those on the *Confidence* questionnaire. Hopefully, the patient ranked these as a "1" – meaning they are confident that they will continue to do these activities. It is important that you talk with the patient about these activities to confirm their ranking for accuracy in your professional judgement.

Next, look on the *Readiness* questionnaire for those activities ranked as a "3." Compare these with the *Confidence* questionnaire to see if any are ranked as a "1" or "2." If so, these activities are the ones that should be strongly considered for implementation in the very near future. These results indicate that the patient is "ready" and "confident" to participate in these lifestyle medicine activities. Using this method may promote self-efficacy which can then boost self-confidence when attempting to implement other lifestyle medicine activities in the future.

Clinical judgment should be used when choosing which lifestyle medicine activities to implement and how many lifestyle medicine activities should be started at any one time. Some research supports the idea that only one lifestyle medicine activity should be started at any time, while other research supports the idea of implementing multiple lifestyle medicine activities at the same time. Additionally, the patient's risk factors and clinical profile may help determine which activities to implement first.

References

1. Lenz TL, Stading JA. Lifestyle modification counseling of patients with dyslipidemias by pharmacists and other health care professionals. J Am Pharm Assoc. 2005;45:709-713.
2. Sebate E. Aherence to long-term therapies: evidence for action. Geneva: World Health Organization, 2003. Available at: http://who.int/chp/knowledge/publications/adherence_full_report.pdf. Accessed December 10, 2012.
3. Bosworth HB. Medication adherence: making the case for increased awareness. National Consumers League. Available at: http://scriptyourfuture.org/wp-content/themes/cons/m/Script_ Your_Future_Briefing_Paper.pdf. Accessed December 10, 2012.
4. Osterberg L, Blaschke T. Adherence to medication. N Engl Med. 2005;353:487-497.
5. Centers for Disease Control and Prevention. The Behavioral Risk Factor Surveillance System. Prevalence and Trends Data. Available at: http://apps.nccd.cdc.gov/brfss/. Accessed December 10, 2012.
6. Mokdad AH, Marks JS, Stroup DF, Gerberding JL. Actual causes of death in the United States, 2000. JAMA. 2004;291:1238-1246.
7. Miller RR, Sales AE, Kopjar B, Fihn SD, Bryson CL. Adherence to heart-healthy behaviors in a sample of the U.S. population. Prev Chronic Dis 2005 April. Available at: URL: http://www.cdc.gov/pcd/issues/2005/apr/04_0115.htm. Accessed on: December 2, 2012.

8. Clark NM, Houle CR. Theoretical models and strategies for improving disease management by patients. In: Shumaker SA, et al., eds. The Handbook for Health Behavior Change, 3rd ed. New York: Springer Publishing Company, 2009:19-38.
9. Prochaska JO, Johnson S, Lee P. The Transtheoretical Model of Behavior Change. In: Shumaker SA, et al., eds. The Handbook for Health Behavior Change, 3rd ed. New York: Springer Publishing Company, 2009:59-84.

3   Physical Activity

Objectives
1. Define physical activity and exercise.
2. Explain the health benefits of physical activity.
3. Recall the current recommendations for physical activity.

Of all the core components of lifestyle medicine, physical activity ranks as one of the most commonly recognized. Most people are aware that physical activity and exercise are good for the body (and mind) and important for achieving overall health. The benefits of exercise have been written about for centuries, but the scientific evidence supporting exercise is less then 75 years old.[1] The first physical activity recommendations from national organizations, such as the American Heart Association, appeared in the 1970's.[1]

"Walking is man's best medicine." Hippocrates, c. 460 BC – c. 370 BC

Many different terms are used when discussing physical activity. It is important to begin our study of physical activity by defining these terms so we have a uniform understanding as we move forward.

Physical Activity. Any bodily movement produced by skeletal muscles that results in energy expenditure.[1] (e.g. walking, biking, lifting pushing, digging, recreation sports)

Physical Inactivity. The lack of any regular pattern of physical activity beyond that required for daily functioning.[1]

Exercise. Purposeful physical activity that is planned or structured and performed with the intent to improve physical fitness. (e.g. walking, jogging, biking, exercise class, swimming, rowing)

Physical Fitness. A state of improved physical condition achieved through participation in one or more of the following activities - cardiorespiratory endurance, muscular strength, muscular endurance, flexibility, and body composition.

Cardiorespiratory Endurance. The ability of the circulatory and respiratory systems to supply fuel and oxygen to the body during sustained physical activity - also called aerobic endurance.

Muscular Strength. The ability of the skeletal muscles to exert force during physical activity.

Muscular Endurance. The ability of the skeletal muscles to sustain performance without undue fatigue during physical activity.

Flexibility. The range of motion around a joint.

Body Composition. The relative amounts of muscle, fat, bone and other major components of the body.[1]

Aerobic Exercise. Activities that raise the heart rate to a consistent level, use large muscle groups, are performed for long periods of time, and are rhythmic in nature.

On many occasions throughout this book, the terms physical activity and exercise will be used. The intent is to not use these terms interchangeably. Physical activity will be used when discussing general bodily movement, such as the concept of "moving more and sitting less." Increased physical activity can be achieved through purposeful exercise, but in several other ways as well. These can include one's job if it is physical in nature, leisure time activities such as sports, recreation and hobbies, and work around the house such as sweeping floors, gardening and mowing. The term exercise will be used when discussing purposeful and planned physical activity with the intent to improve physical fitness. It is important to note that a general increase in physical activity and increased exercise have both shown to prevent many types of diseases and chronic conditions.

Health Benefits of Physical Activity and Exercise

As stated in the introduction of this chapter, the scientific evidence supporting the benefits of physical activity has been studied for about the last 75 years. In 2008, the United States Department of Health and Human Services (USDHHS) published their most recent version of the physical activity guidelines entitled, *2008 Physical Activity Guidelines for Americans*.[1] These guidelines provide an evidence-based review of the many benefits of physical activity and are listed below.[1] Note that these benefits are experienced with regular and consist participation in physical activity. The specific amounts of physical activity/exercise needed will be discussed in the next section.

- *All Cause Mortality*
    - 30% decrease in death from any cause
    - life expectancy at age 20 increases between 2.4 and 5.5 years over a lifetime[2]

- *Cardiorespiratory Health*
    - 20% to 35% lower risk for coronary heart disease (CHD), cardiovascular disease (CVD) and stroke
    - prevent and treat hypertension and atherogenic dyslipidemia
    - improve cardiorespiratory fitness

- *Metabolic Health*
    - prevent and treat type 2 diabetes mellitus and metabolic syndrome (30% to 40% lower risk of each)

- *Energy Balance*
    - weight maintenance, weight loss and weight maintenance following weight loss

- *Musculoskeletal Health*
    - increase muscle strength
    - improve symptoms associated with osteoarthritis, rheumatoid arthritis, and fibromyalgia
    - improve bone density by 1% to 2%
    - reduce risk for hip fractures by 36% to 68%

- *Functional Health*
    - 30% risk reduction for the prevention or delay in functional abilities in older adults
    - reduces risk for fall in older adults

•*Cancer*
  ◦30% lower risk for colon cancer
  ◦20% lower risk for breast cancer

•*Mental Health*
  ◦20% to 30% lower risk for depression, anxiety and dementia
  ◦reduces stress

•*Other*
  ◦improves health related quality of life
  ◦improves sleep

Fitness vs. Fatness

For most individuals, obesity is an undeniable risk factor for developing CVD and other chronic conditions. However, research shows that physical activity may be able to negate much of the risks associated with obesity. In a meta-analysis published in 1999, researchers showed that individuals who are physically active appear to be protected against the health risks associated with obesity - namely CVD, CHD, hypertension, type 2 diabetes and all-cause mortality.[3] The review also showed that obese individuals who are active have lower morbidity and mortality rates compared with normal weight individuals who are sedentary. Physical inactivity and low fitness levels appear to be as important of a risk factor as obesity.[3]

Components of an Exercise Program

Fundamentally, there are five components to an exercise program. Participation in each of the components is not necessary in order to advance one's health. However, participating in all five components on a regular basis will provide a balanced fitness approach and promote safety and injury prevention.

1. **Warm-up**. The warm-up period, prior to participating in the actual exercise session, is carried out to safely transition the body from a resting state to an exercising state. A proper warm-up will get the body ready for exercise by augmenting blood flow to the working muscles and the cardiorespiratory system, increasing metabolic rate and by helping stretch the muscles. The warm-up will also decrease

injury risk and improve exercise performance. The warm-up period should begin with 5 to 10 minutes of stretching exercises of the major muscle groups followed by 5 to 10 minutes of progressive, low intensity aerobic activity that will sufficiently raise the heart rate.[4] For most individuals, walking is a good warm-up activity but it can also simply be the same activity as planned in the actual exercise session, but at a lower intensity.

2. **Aerobic Conditioning**. The USDHHS *2008 Physical Activity Guidelines for Americans* provides the following recommendations for adults:

Accumulate a minimum of 150 minutes (2 hours and 30 minutes) of moderate-intensity activity each week.

OR

Accumulate a minimum of 75 minutes (1 hour and 15 minutes) of vigorous-intensity activity each week.

OR

Accumulate an equivalent combination of moderate- and vigorous-intensity activity each week.

There appears to be a well founded dose-response relationship between aerobic exercise and the health benefits listed above. For most of the physical activity health benefits, the amount of exercise required to obtain these benefits appears to be similar - 150 minutes per week of moderate-intensity aerobic activity.[1] The scheduling of the exercise sessions, however, can vary and be customized to individual needs. The only stipulation is that each exercise session must be at least 10 minutes in duration to obtain the benefits.[1] The guidelines also report that additional health benefits can be obtained from up to 300 minutes per week of moderate-intensity or 150 minutes per week of vigorous-intensity aerobic exercise. Lastly, it is important to note that the minimum amount of aerobic exercise required for effective weight loss, may be more than suggested above by the USDHHS. This will be covered in further details in *Chapter 9, Overweight and Obesity*.

✓ **Fast Fact:** Only 20.7% of adults meet the federal guidelines for physical activity.

---

3. **Resistance (Muscle-Strengthening) Training**. The USDHHS *2008 Physical Activity Guidelines for Americans* provides the following recommendations for adults:

> On 2 or more days per week, resistance training exercises should be performed on all major muscle groups
> (i.e. legs, hips, back, abdomen, chest, shoulders, and arms)

The number of repetitions and sets of repetitions of each exercise varies depending on the desired outcomes. In general, lifting heavier weight for fewer repetitions (1 to 6) will promote muscular strength. Lifting moderate weight for 8 to 12 repetitions will promote muscular strength and size (especially in men). Lastly, lifting lighter weight for 15 to 20 repetitions will promote muscular endurance. It is recommended that adults lift moderate or lighter weights with the appropriate repetitions and older adults lift lighter weights with higher repetitions to promote strength and endurance while preventing injury.[1] It is recommended that proper training on exercise technique should be taught by a trained professional before beginning a resistance training program to ensure the exercises are performed safely, properly and in the correct order.

4. **Stretching**. Stretching is important for an exercise program because it allows for increases in musculoskeletal function, balance, and agility. It also improves functional ability - the ability to perform activities of daily living. Most importantly, however, stretching is important for injury prevention. Stretching exercises should be performed on all major joints such as the hips, back, shoulders, knees, upper trunk and neck regions.[4] Stretching should incorporate slow movements that are sustained for 10 to 30 seconds. A minimum of 4 repetitions for each muscle group should be performed on a minimum of 2 to 3 days per week. The degree of stretch should be done smoothly without bounce and should not cause pain, but mild discomfort is acceptable. Stretching activities can be incorporated with the warm-up and/or cool-down activities, but may be easier to perform if done so during the cool-down.

5. **Cool-Down**. The purpose of the cool-down period is to return the body to its pre-exercise state through a gradual decrease in heart rate, blood pressure, and respiration. It also facilitates the dissipation of body heat. A proper cool-down period will decrease the possibility of post-exercise hypotension (low blood pressure) and dizziness.[4] The recommendations for the cool-down are the same as those for the warm-up, but performed in reverse order.

Writing an Exercise Prescription

Most people think of a prescription as instructions from a physician on how to take a medication. However, a prescription is not limited to medications and by definition is simply a set of instructions. Lifestyle medicine activities can be used similarly and in conjunction with medications to treat chronic conditions, and as a result, can be prescribed. The purpose of an exercise prescription is to provide an individual with a specific and personalized set of instructions on how to carry out an exercise program that can promote health, enhance physical fitness, prevent and manage chronic conditions, and limit the risk of injury.[4] There are six essential parts of an exercise prescription. These six components can be applied to all individuals regardless of age, fitness level, exercise experience or chronic condition. Exercise prescriptions should be developed with careful consideration to each individual's current health status, risk factors, personal goals, physical activity preferences, previous exercise experiences, and behavioral characteristics. It may also be important to work with other members of the individual's health care team when writing an exercise prescription to ensure all pertinent information is considered.

1. **Personal Goals**. As with any prescription, involving the individual for whom the prescription is being written is an important and often overlooked step. Each individual should have a personalized set of exercise goals, and as a result, an individually specific exercise prescription. No one exercise prescription is appropriate for all individuals. Some people may have several goals while others may only have a few. The goals should be prioritized and addressed as the most important goal(s) receiving the greatest amount of effort and attention. Working directly with the individual to identify and develop realistic and achievable goals can evoke greater program accountability and, as a result, lead to greater program success.

33

2. **Mode** (type of activity). Several factors come into play when choosing the type of activity. The most important factor may be the personal preferences of the patient. Activities that are enjoyable to the individual will more likely lead to greater program adherence. Exercise adherence may be the single most important factor leading to successful outcomes resulting from an exercise prescription. The type of activity must also match the physical abilities of the individual. For example, recommending jogging to someone who is sedentary with osteoarthritis of the knees would not be a wise choice because it may be painful and can possibly lead to injury and poor adherence. It may be better to suggest that this individual participate in activities that are non-weight bearing, at least initially. On the other hand, a person who is at risk for osteoporosis may benefit a great deal from participating in weight bearing activities as they have been shown to build bone and increase bone strength.

3. **Intensity**. In the *2008 Physical Activity Guidelines for Americans*, it is recommended for all adults to accumulate at least 150 minutes per week of moderate-intensity aerobic activity.[1] Intensity refers to the workload of a particular exercise or activity. All physical activities are generally placed into one of three intensity categories: light, moderate or vigorous. Activities are placed into each category according to their workload, which is measured in METs (Metabolic EquivalenTs). METs are a useful and convenient way to describe the intensity of a variety of activities.[4]

•1 MET = the amount of energy the body uses each minute while resting quietly
•Less than 3 METs = light-intensity activities
•3 to 6 METs = moderate-intensity activities
•More than 6 METs = vigorous-intensity activities

A few examples of activities within each category is listed here. A more compete list of examples can be found in reference 5 of this chapter or at http://www.cdc.gov/nccdphp/dnpa/physical/.../PA _Intensity_table_2_1.pdf

Light
 Walking, 2 mph (2.5 METs)
 Golfing, with a cart (2.5 METs)
 Dancing, ballroom, slow (2.9 METs)

Moderate
 Bicycling, level surface (4.0 METs)
 Golfing, carrying clubs (4.5 METs)
 Walking, 15 minutes/mile (5.0 METs)

Vigorous
 Swimming laps, moderate pace (7.0 METs)
 Bicycling, 12-13 mph (8.0 METs)
 Running, 9 minutes/mile (11.0 METs)

✓ **Fast Fact:** When using a pedometer, walking 100 steps/min is considered a moderate-intensity pace.

Besides picking the appropriate type of activity to match the desired intensity level, it is also a good idea to monitor the body's response to the activity while exercising. Monitoring the body's response can help ensure that the appropriate level of intensity is being achieved. It can also serve as a safety check to ensure the type of activity and intensity level are appropriate for each individual.

There are several ways to monitor intensity while exercising. Each of the methods is based on the physiological response of the heart and lungs as a result of the increased workload. As the body experiences an increased workload from exercise, the heart rate and respiratory rate increase in response to the need for more oxygenation in the blood and muscle tissues. One method of measuring exercise intensity is to simply measure the heart rate during the exercise session. This method is called Target Heart Rate (THR) and a great deal of research has been conducted on this method. Although THR is a valid method to measure exercise intensity, it is difficult for some individuals to understand and calculate. Further information regarding THR can be found at http://www.cdc.gov/physicalactivity/everyone/measuring/heartrate.html.

An easier method of measuring exercise intensity, although less exact, is the Talk Test. The Talk Test method involves simply self-monitoring the ability to carry a conversation while exercising. As a rule of thumb, a person participating in an activity at a light intensity level will be able to sing while doing the activity.[6] Someone active at a moderate-intensity level should be able to carry on a conversation while participating in the activity, but will likely not be able to sing. Lastly, a person participating in an activity that is considered vigorous will be too winded and out of breath to carry on a conversation. At the vigorous-intensity level a person will not be able to say more than a few words without pausing for a breath.[6] This method of measuring exercise intensity is easy for patients to understand and measure themselves without a great deal of assistance from others.

4. **Duration**. The duration portion of an exercise prescription is a measure of the length (usually measured in minutes) of the exercise session. The duration of an activity is inversely related to the intensity of the activity. Light-intensity activities can be sustained for a longer duration and vigorous-intensity activities can only be sustained for short durations of time due to the greater oxygen requirements of the muscle. The *2008 Physical Activity Guidelines for Americans* recommends a total weekly duration of at least 150 minutes at a moderate-intensity with each bout of exercise lasting at least 10 minutes in duration.[1] Intermittent bouts of physical activity may be very useful and practical for certain individuals. Intermittent bouts of activity have been shown to improve exercise adherence in individuals who are not accustomed to physical activity and may be safer for patients who are severely deconditioned because it allows for more frequent rest and recovery until continuous exercise can be sustained.

✓ **Fast Fact:** When using a pedometer, averaging 7000 steps per day for 7 days is equal to achieving 150 minutes of physical activity per week.

---

5. **Frequency**. Frequency refers to the number of days per week an individual will partake in physical activity. This is a good time to again make the distinction between physical activity and exercise. Physical activity refers to all activity and emphasizes the "move more, sit less" principle. Therefore, the frequency of physical activity

should be daily and ideally, several times daily. Exercise frequency recommendations, however, are not as prescriptive as they once were and are, in fact, not even mentioned in the general guidelines statement. Rather, the recommendation leaves room for a personalized exercise program to maximize program adherence. Some individuals may want to exercise for 30 minutes/day on 5 days/week to achieve their total of 150 minutes. Others, however may exercise in shorter bouts more often or longer bouts on fewer days per week. The accumulated time of both increased overall physical activity and exercise is ultimately more important then the specific schedule by which it is achieved.

6. **Rate of Progression**. An exercise prescription should be continually evaluated for its effectiveness at achieving each persons goals. When designing an exercise prescription, the patient and health care provider should have a general plan for how the program progresses to meet the stated goals. Some individuals may need to start with low levels of exercise and progress slowly, while others can progress more aggressively. It is important to understand that not all individuals will be able (or willing) to achieve the current recommendations for physical activity. The goal for everyone, however, should be consistency of participation with gradual movement towards the recommendations.

Physical activity progression is generally thought of in three separate stages; initial, improvement, and maintenance.[4] The initial stage is lower in intensity, duration and frequency to decrease the risk of injury and muscle soreness. Adherence to the program is one of the primary goals of the phase. The intensity can start at light and progress to moderate and the duration can begin as low as 5 minutes but progress to 30 minutes by the end of four weeks. This phase usually lasts up to four weeks. Deconditioned individuals should be permitted more time to adapt to each stage within the program.[4]

The second stage is called the improvement stage.[4] The goal of this stage is to make gradual increases in duration, frequency and intensity, with emphasis on duration and frequency to improve cardiorespiratory endurance. This stage will typically last four to five months.[4]

The third stage is the maintenance stage where long-term maintenance and adherence to the physical activity program is the main goal.[4] During this stage, the major long-term goals of the physical activity program should be evaluated with the possibility of reassigning new goals for ones that have been accomplished.

Energy Expenditure

Physical activity, and especially purposeful exercise, is an important component for controlling body weight because of its effect on direct and indirect energy expenditure. The amount of total direct energy expended while performing an activity becomes important when designing a weight loss program. This can be estimated using a simple formula involving the MET level of the activity.[4]

Calculating the caloric expenditure of any physical activity can be estimated, but it is not an exact science. Several factors may influence the energy expenditure of an activity, such as skill, coordination and exercise efficiency as well as the variable intensities that may exist within an individual activity.[4] One method to approximate the caloric expenditure of a specific activity uses the formula:

$$(METs \times 3.5 \times body\ weight\ in\ kg)/200 = kcal/min$$

Let's use an example. An exercise prescription designed for a 51 year old male weighting 102 kg recommends that the he walk at a 15 min/mile pace for 30 minutes per day, three times per week. Walking at this intensity has a corresponding MET value of 5.0. Using the energy expenditure formula above we can calculate this individuals caloric expenditure from this specific exercise prescription:

$$(5.0 \times 3.5 \times 102)/200 = 8.9\ calories/min$$

This individual will expend almost 9 calories per minute or about 267 calories per exercise session (8.9 kcal/min x 30 min = 267 calories/day) while walking. In addition, he will expend about 801 calories per week (267 kcal/day x 3 day/week) as a result of the exercise prescription.

Injury Prevention

The first objective for health care providers when designing an exercise prescription is to provide a program that is safe and will not harm the individual. The most common risks associated with physical activity are related to injury of the musculoskeletal system, which includes the bones, joints, tendons and muscles.[7] Sedentary individuals who begin an exercise program and experience pain from an injury or undue muscle soreness are not likely to be adherent to the program. Musculoskeletal injuries can be minimized through gradual increases in intensity, duration and frequency, proper warm-up and cool-down with stretching, and by avoiding excessive amounts of activity at one time.[7] Therefore, patients with little experience participating in physical activity should begin slowly by incorporating only a few minutes of physical activity into their day and gradually increase duration as their bodies adjust.

Cardiac events can occur in certain individuals during vigorous exercise, but the incidence of these events is low. The American Heart Association (AHA) recommends that physicians not overestimate the risks of exercise because the benefits of habitual physical activity outweigh the risks.[8] However, the American College of Sports Medicine and the AHA recommend that individuals with known or suspected cardiovascular, pulmonary or metabolic disease obtain medical clearance before beginning a vigorous exercise program.[4] In addition, it would be prudent for health care providers prescribing exercise to contact an individual patient's physician and health care team to effectively communicate the exercise program. This keeps the physician and team informed of the patient's overall health and can be another source of encouragement and motivation for the patient to continue the program.

Summary Points

●Physical activity is any bodily movement that results in energy expenditure while exercise is purposeful physical activity that is planned or structured and performed with the intent to improve physical fitness.
●Benefits of physical activity and exercise include lower mortality, improved cardiorespiratory health, improved metabolic health, more effective energy balance, greater musculoskeletal and functional health, lower risk for certain cancers, and an improved quality of life.

●The USDHHS recommends a minimum of 150 minutes/week of moderate intensity physical activity.
●The components of an exercise program include warm-up, aerobic conditioning, resistance training, stretching, and cool-down.
●The essential components of an exercise prescription include personal goals, mode, intensity, duration, frequency, and rate of progression.
●The most commonly experienced injuries from physical activity and exercise are related to the musculoskeletal system.

Test Your Knowledge

1. Planned and structured activity performed for the purposes of improving fitness is the definition for:

a. physical activity
b. exercise
c. cardiorespiratory endurance
d. flexibility

2. All of the following are essential components of an exercise prescription EXCEPT:

a. personal goals
b. type of activity
c. intensity
d. family history
e. frequency

3. The metabolic equivalent (MET) level for moderate-intensity physical activity is:

a. 1 to 3
b. 3 to 6
c. 6 to 9
d. 9 or greater

References

1. Physical Activity Guidelines Advisory Committee. Physical Activity Guidelines Advisory Committee Report, 2008. Washington, DC: US. Department of Health and Human Services, 2008.
2. Janssen I, Carson V, Lee I, Katzmarzyk PT, Blair SN. Years of life gained due to leisure-time physical activity in the U.S. Am J Prev Med 2013;44(1):23-29.
3. Blair SN, Brodney S. Effects of physical activity and obesity on morbidity and mortality: current evidence and research issues. Med Sci Sports Exerc 1999;31(Suppl):S646-S662.
4. American College of Sports Medicine. Guidelines for Exercise Testing and Prescription, 8th ed. Baltimore: Wolters Kluwer Lippincott Williams & Wilkins, 2010.
5. Ainsworth BE, Haskell MC, Whitt ML, Irwin AM, Swartz SJ, Strath WL, et al. Compendium of physical activities: an update of activity codes and MET intensities. Medicine and Science in Sport and Exercise 2000;32(9) Suppl S498-S516.
6. Centers for Disease Control and Prevention. Measuring physical activity intensity. Available at: http://www.cdc.gov/physicalactivity/everyone/measuring/index.html. Accessed on January 9, 2013.
7. Fletcher GF, Balady SN, Blair SN, et al. Benefits and recommendations for physical activity programs for all Americans. A statement for health professionals by the Committee for Exercise and Cardiac Rehabilitation of the Council of Clinical Cardiology, American Heart Association. Circulation 1996;94:857-862.
8. American College of Sports Medicine, American Heart Association. Exercise and acute cardiovascular events: placing the risk into perspective. Med Sci Sports Exerc 2007;39(5):886-897.

4   Healthy Eating

Objectives
1. Explain the relationship between healthy eating and chronic disease prevention and management.
2. Outline the key recommendations of the *2010 Dietary Guidelines for Americans*.
3. Summarize the three classes of macronutrients.

Eating is a fundamental and necessary part of life. Along with sleep, it is the only other lifestyle activity covered in this book that is required each and everyday day for all persons to sustain life. Healthy eating is necessary for proper growth, development, and well-being throughout an individual's lifespan. Conversely, unhealthy eating can be a significant contributor to many preventable chronic diseases such as cardiovascular disease, cancer, obesity, and diabetes. The belief that eating healthy is an important part of life has been known for centuries.

> "If we could give every individual the right amount of nourishment and exercise, not too little and not too much, we would have found the safest way to health." Hippocrates, c. 460 BC – c. 370 BC

The subject of healthy eating can be divided into two separate topics: quality of food consumption and quantity of food consumption. Each of these topics should be discussed separately so that a distinction can be made when learning about the fundamentals of lifestyle medicine. This chapter will focus on both with further discussion of quantity covered in *Chapter 9, Overweight and Obesity*. One of the basic concepts to be cognizant of while reading this chapter is the notion that everyone must eat. It is different then our discussions about tobacco and alcohol use where we can devise a program to quit. We cannot simply quit eating to improve health. Rather, developing a positive relationship with food so that a healthy coexistence becomes a reality is necessary for everyone in order to obtain optimal health and resist disease.

Healthy Eating and Chronic Disease

A growing body of scientific evidence demonstrates that healthy eating, along with adequate physical activity, may help reduce the risk for chronic diseases.[1] Among the most significant of these chronic conditions is excess body weight. Apart from this, however, unhealthy eating and physical inactivity are associated with major causes of morbidity and mortality. These include cardiovascular disease (CVD), hypertension, type 2 diabetes, osteoporosis, and some types of cancers.[1] More specifically, excessive sodium and alcohol consumption, insufficient potassium intake, and overweight and obesity are all related to healthy eating and have been shown to increase blood pressure.[1] Dietary factors are associated with increased risk of some types of cancer, including breast (post menopausal), endometrial, colon, kidney, mouth, and esophageal.[1]

Dietary Guidelines for Americans, 2010

By law, *Dietary Guidelines for Americans* is reviewed, updated and published every 5 years.[1] The U.S. Department of Agriculture (USDA) and the U.S. Department of Health and Human Services (HHS) jointly create each edition and the document is generally referred to as the "Dietary Guidelines." The *Dietary Guidelines for Americans, 2010* is intended for Americans ages 2 and older, including those at increased risk for chronic disease.[1] It provides recommendations that encompass two overarching concepts:

•Maintain calorie balance over time to achieve
and sustain a healthy weight.
•Focus on consuming nutrient-dense foods and beverages.

The prevalence of overweight and obesity continue to increase in America and as a result, the *2010 Dietary Guidelines* focuses a great deal of recommendations on this issue. In addition, many of the recommendations mention physical activity as an important component of a healthy lifestyle, in particular a healthy body weight. A concerted effort has been made by the HHS to emphasize the importance of both the *2008 Physical Activity Guidelines for Americans* (discussed in the previous chapter) and the *2010 Dietary Guidelines for Americans* and that they should be used together to combat chronic diseases and achieve greater overall health.

There are 4 Key Recommendations that are discussed in detail within the *2010 Dietary Guidelines*. To get the full benefit, individuals should carry out the guideline recommendations in their entirety as part of an overall healthy eating plan.[1] The following is a summary of the 4 Key Recommendations as they are stated in the *2010 Dietary Guidelines*:[1]

1. **Balancing calories to manage weight.**

•Prevent and/or reduce overweight and obesity through improved eating and physical activity behaviors.
•Control total calorie intake to manage body weight. For people who are overweight or obese, this will mean consuming fewer calories from foods and beverages.
•Increase physical activity and reduce time spent in sedentary behaviors.
•Maintain appropriate calorie balance during each stage of life - childhood, adolescence, adulthood, pregnancy and breastfeeding, and older age.

2. **Foods and food components to reduce.**

•Reduce dietary sodium intake to less than 2,300 mg per day. Further reduce intake to 1,500 mg per day for persons who are 51 and older and those of any age who are African American or have hypertension, diabetes, or chronic kidney disease. The 1,500 mg per day recommendation applies to about half of the U.S. population, including children, and the majority of adults.
•Consume less than 10% of calories from saturated fatty acids. Replace with monounsaturated and polyunsaturated fatty acids.
•Consume less than 300 mg per day of dietary cholesterol.
•Keep trans fatty acid consumption as low as possible by limiting foods that contain synthetic sources of trans fats, such as partially hydrogenated oils, and by limiting other solid fats.
•Reduce intake of calories from solid fats and added sugars.
•Limit consumption of foods that contain refined grains, especially refined grain foods that contain solid fats, added sugars, and sodium.
•If alcohol is consumed, it should be consumed in moderation.

3. **Foods and nutrients to increase**. Individuals should meet the following recommendations as part of a healthy eating plan while staying within their calorie needs:

•Increase vegetable and fruit intake.
•Eat a variety of vegetables - especially dark green, red and orange colored, beans and peas.
•Consume at least 1/2 of all grains as whole grains. Increase whole grain intake by replacing refined grains with whole grains.
•Increase intake of fat-free or low-fat milk and milk products, such as milk, yogurt, cheese, or fortified soy beverages.
•Choose a variety of protein foods, which include seafood, lean meat and poultry, eggs, beans and peas, soy products, and unsalted nuts and seeds.
•Increase the amount and variety of seafood consumed by choosing seafood in place of some meat and poultry.
•Replace protein foods that are higher in solid fats with choices that are lower in solid fats and calories and/or are sources of oils.
•Use oils to replace solid fats when possible.
•Choose foods that provide more potassium, dietary fiber, calcium, and vitamin D, which are nutrients of concern in American diets. These foods include vegetables, fruits, whole grains, and milk and milk products.
•Individuals 50 years and older should consume foods fortified with vitamin B12, such as fortified cereals, or dietary supplements.

4. **Building healthy eating patterns.**

•Select an eating pattern that satisfies nutrient needs over time at an appropriate calorie level.
•Account for all foods and beverages consumed and assess how they fit within a total healthy eating plan.
•Follow food safety recommendations when preparing and eating foods to reduce the risk of food-born illnesses.

Nutrition Fundamentals

Food As Energy

The fundamental purpose of eating is to provide the body with adequate amounts of energy needed to perform many different metabolic and physiologic functions.[1] The energy that is gained from the food we eat is expressed as calories. A calorie is commonly abbreviated as either "C" or "kcal."

Energy obtained from food can be derived from three major sources: carbohydrate, fat, and protein. These three sources are collectively known as macronutrients. Calories can also be obtained from the consumption of alcohol. This source, however, contains little nutritional value outside of its contribution of calories to the diet. A one-gram consumption of each of these sources results in the following number of calories:[2]

- 1 gram carbohydrate = 4 calories
- 1 gram fat = 9 calories
- 1 gram protein = 4 calories
- 1 gram alcohol = 7 calories

Carbohydrates

The *Dietary Guidelines* recommend that adults consume the majority of their calories from carbohydrate sources. Of the total caloric needs required each day, 45% to 65% of them should come from carbohydrates.[1] The *Dietary Guidelines* refers to carbohydrates as grains. The key to healthy eating with grains is choosing the right type to consume. Not all grains are created equal. Although most Americans generally eat enough total grains, most of the grains consumed are refined grains rather than whole grains.

There are three major categories of carbohydrate: simple carbohydrates, complex carbohydrates, and dietary fiber.[2] Simple carbohydrates are often called sugars and can be found naturally in fruits, vegetables and milk products but can also be man-made such as refined sugars like high fructose corn syrup. Complex carbohydrates are also called starches. Complex carbohydrates can come from whole-grain products as well as refined grains.

Whole grains are the preferred type of carbohydrate and are a source of nutrients like iron, magnesium, selenium, B vitamins, and dietary fiber. Whole grains can vary in their dietary fiber content. Some evidence suggests that whole grain intake may reduce the risk for cardiovascular disease and is associated with lower body weight. Some evidence, although limited, suggests that consuming whole grains is associated with a lower incidence of type 2 diabetes.

> ✓ **Fast Fact:** Less than 5% of Americans consume the minimum recommended amount of whole-grains.

It may be helpful to explain the difference between whole grains, refined grains and enriched grains. Whole grains contain the entire grain seed, usually called the kernel. The kernel consists of three components-the bran, germ, and endosperm. Some examples of whole-grain ingredients include buckwheat, bulgar, millet, oatmeal, quinoa, rolled oats, brown or wild rice, whole-grain barley, whole rye, and whole wheat.[1]

Refined grains have been milled to remove the bran and germ from the grain. This is done to improve both the texture and shelf-life of the product. However, it also removes some of the nutrients such as iron, many of the B vitamins and dietary fiber.[1] Most refined grain products will have the B vitamins and iron added or fortified back into the product. These are called enriched grains. Refined and enriched grains most often contain lower dietary fiber compared with whole-grain products.

Dietary fiber is a non-digestible form of carbohydrates and lignin and naturally occurs in plants.[1] Eating sources rich in dietary fiber helps provide a feeling of fullness when eating and can help promote healthy laxation.[1] Dietary fiber that naturally occurs in foods may help reduce the risk of cardiovascular disease, obesity and type 2 diabetes. The recommended daily intake of dietary fiber is 14 grams per 1000 calories consumed.[1] For women, this is approximately 25 grams per day and for men this is about 38 grams per day. Some of the best sources of dietary fiber include beans and peas, such as navy beans, split peas, lentils, pinto beans and black beans.[1] Other good sources of dietary fiber include fruits, vegetables, whole grains and nuts.

✓ **Fast Fact:** On average in America, adults consume about 15 grams of fiber per day.

Simple sugars are found in natural products such as fruit (fructose) and milk (lactose). However, the majority of sugar intake in the typical American diet comes from sugar added to foods during processing or preparation.[1] The "added sugars" further sweeten the flavor and improve the looks of some products as well as enhance preservation.[1] Examples of added sugars include high fructose corn syrup, white sugar, brown sugar, corn syrup, corn syrup solids, fructose sweetener, liquid fructose, honey, molasses, anhydrous dextrose, and crystal dextrose.[1] The most significant sources of added sugars in the American diet come from soda, energy drinks, and sport-drinks.[1]

✓ **Fast Fact:** Added sugars contribute an average of 16% of the total calories in American diets.

Protein

The *Dietary Guidelines* recommend that adults consume 10% to 35% of their total calories from protein food sources.[1] Proteins are an important food source because they help to regulate human metabolism by taking part in the formation of almost all enzymes and several hormones that control physiologic functions, such as regulation of the blood clotting system, acid-base balance, and the development of the immune system.[2] Proteins play a key role in providing the structural basis and nutrients needed for most tissues in the body.

Sources for quality protein can be found in both plant and animal foods. Coincidentally, good food sources for protein are similar to foods that contain fiber, such as dry beans, lentils, peas, nuts, seeds and processed soy products. Other sources of protein include meat, poultry, seafood, and eggs. Meat and poultry sources should be lean or low-fat and nuts should be unsalted. The fats that are contained in meat, poultry, and eggs are considered solid fats while the fats in seafoods, nuts and seeds are considered oils (discussed in the next section). Therefore, the recommended sources of protein comes from beans, peas, nuts, seeds and seafood because they have the preferred type of fats as well as a good source of dietary fiber. Note that beans and peas are considered part of this group as well as the vegetable group.[1]

Fats

Dietary fats and oils are an essential part of a healthful diet. The type of fat and the total amount of fat consumed, however, do make a difference when considering the health benefits. Dietary fats are found in both plant and animal foods. Fats supply calories and essential fatty acids. Fats also help in the absorption of the fat-soluble vitamins A, D, E, and K.[1] The *Dietary Guidelines* recommend that 20% to 35% of the total calories consumed each day by adults should come from fats.

Fatty acids are categorized as being saturated, monounsaturated, or polyunsaturated. A combination of all three categories is referred to as fats. Trans fatty acids are unsaturated fatty acids that are structurally different from the more predominant unsaturated fatty acids that occur naturally in plant foods. It is important to understand that when discussing the risk of cardiovascular disease associated with dietary fat intake, the type of fatty acid is more important than the total amount of fat consumed. As a general rule, animal sources of fat tend to be higher in saturated fats (with the exception of seafood), whereas plant sources of fat tend to he higher in monounsaturated and/or polyunsaturated fats.[1]

Saturated fatty acids are physiologically necessary for overall health, however, the body makes more than it needs for these physiological requirements.[1] Therefore, it is not necessary to consume saturated fats in the diet. Saturated fats are generally solid at room temperature and are often referred to as solid fats. The *Dietary Guidelines* recommends that American adults consume less than 10% of their total calories from saturated fats. Saturated fatty acids have been shown to increase total and LDL-cholesterol levels. Replacing saturated fats with monounsaturated and/or polyunsaturated fats is associated with low blood cholesterol levels, and therefore a lower risk for cardiovascular disease.[1] Reducing the amount to less than 7% of total calories can reduce this risk even further. The most significant sources of saturated fats in the American diet is from cheese, pizza, grain-based deserts, dairy-based deserts, chicken, sausage, franks, bacon and ribs.[1]

✓ **Fast Fact:** Solid fats contribute an average of 19% of the total calories in the American diet.

Fats with a high percentage of monounsaturated and polyunsaturated fatty acids are usually liquid at room temperature and are referred to as oils.[1] Because oils are a concentrated source of calories (9 kcal/gm), Americans should replace solid fats with oils, rather than add oils to their diet.[1] Oils are naturally found in foods such as olives, nuts, avocados, and seafood.[1] They are also extracted from plants such as canola, corn, olive, peanut, safflower, soybean, and sunflower plants. For nutritional purposes, coconut oil, palm kernel oil and palm oil are high in saturated fatty acids and should be considered solid fats. Likewise, partially hydrogenated oils contain trans fatty acids and should be considered solid fats.[1]

Individual Calorie Needs

The total number of calories a person needs each day varies depending on a number of factors, including the person's age, gender, height, weight, and level of physical activity. Knowing one's daily caloric intake may be useful in determining whether the calories that a person eats and drinks are appropriate in relation to the number of calories needed each day to perform physical activity and to control weight.

It is easy to calculate the number of calories that an individual needs on a daily basis. There are several charts and formulas available that can estimate this value. However, it can be very difficult to estimate the number of calories that are actually consumed throughout day in order to compare this to what is required. Rather than counting calories, the best (and easiest) way to assess whether an individual is eating the appropriate number of calories is to monitor body weight and adjust calorie intake and participation in physical activity based on changes in body weight over time.[1] This topic will be covered in greater detail in *Chapter 9, Obesity*. More information is available on calculating individual caloric requirements in the *Dietary Guidelines* website which can be found at: http://www.cnpp.usda.gov/.[1] An alternate method to counting calories is presented below in "Practical Application Tool" and in Toolbox E.

Water

Water contains no calories and therefore, provides no energy. However, water is considered the most essential nutrient for the human body. Most other nutrients needed by the body can only work if adequate amounts of water are present.[2] Water is essential for food digestion, for normal metabolism, and for the regulation of body temperature. In addition, water carries electrolytes that are essential to numerous physiologic processes. The recommended intake of water for adult males and females aged 19 and older is 3.7 and 2.7 liters per day, respectively.[3]

✓ **Fast Fact:** About 20% of our total daily water intake comes from the food we eat.[2]

The *Dietary Guidelines* conclude that the combination of thirst and normal drinking behavior, especially the consumption of fluids with meals, is sufficient to maintain adequate amounts of fluid within the body.[1] Those individuals who are healthy and have sufficient access to fluid consume enough water to satisfy their needs. In conditions in which the environmental temperature is hotter than normal or during physical activity, water intake should be higher.[1] The American College of Sports Medicine (ACSM) recommends drinking 17 ounces of water approximately two hours prior to exercising to achieve adequate hydration during the exercise period.[3]

Summary Points

• Unhealthy eating can be a significant contributor to many preventable chronic diseases such as cardiovascular disease, cancer, obesity, and diabetes.

• The *2010 Dietary Guidelines for Americans* emphasizes: (1) maintaining calorie balance over time to achieve and sustain a healthy weight; and (2) a focus on consuming nutrient-dense foods and beverages.

• Most of the total calorie consumption should come from carbohydrates (grains) sources, particularly whole-grains.

• Added sugar, solid fats and sodium should have limited consumption.

• Caloric needs are individual and should be continually evaluated.

• Physical activity and healthy eating should both be emphasized as part of a healthy lifestyle.

Test Your Knowledge

1. One gram of fat is equal to _____ calories.

a. 4
b. 6
c. 9
d. 10

2. The recommended percentage range of total calories that should come from carbohydrate intake is:

a. less than 10%
b. 20-35%
c. 45-65%
d. greater than 75%

3. Females 19 years of age and older should consume approximately _____ liters of water per day.

a. 1.7
b. 2.7
c. 3.7
d. 4.7

Practical Application Tools

Nutrition and Physical Activity Diary. Research has shown that people who make a habit of writing down what they eat are more health conscious about the type of food they are eating as well as how much they eat. Additionally, people who use a food diary have been shown to lose almost twice as much weight as those who do not use a food diary. Likewise, recording the type and quantity of daily physical activity increases personal awareness about exercise and daily activity habits. The purpose of a nutrition and physical activity diary is to increase awareness about the type, amount, and frequency of food that is consumed throughout the day, as well as the amount of physical activity and exercise performed. Toolbox D provides an example of a nutrition and physical activity diary that can be used on a daily basis to help track personal eating and physical activity habits.

Hunger/Fullness Scale. It is no secret that excess body weight has become a major public health concern. Most people are overweight because of too little physical activity combined with too much food. Over the past several decades our culture has developed in such a way that makes it difficult for us to adequately control how much food we eat. Portion control is one of the most difficult of all the healthy lifestyle activities.

A common question from many people trying to lose weight goes something like this, "Why do I continue to eat when my body has consumed enough calories for the energy I need to live?" The complete answer to this question is complex, but believe it or not, our bodies do send us signals to tell us when we have had enough food. We are all born with the ability to self-regulate how much food we eat. Unfortunately, most of us do not pay attention to our body's natural fullness signals. True portion control is a very natural act that comes simply from listening to our bodies.

The first step to being successful at portion control-the natural way, is to eat more slowly. It takes approximately 15 to 20 minutes for our bodies to tell us that we have eaten enough food. But, the average American eats a meal in less than 10 minutes. The next step is to pay attention to our body's signals that tell us when we are truly hungry and when we are full enough. True signals of hunger include a feeling of an empty stomach, growling noises, or even headache, irritability, tiredness, weakness, dizziness and shakiness when significant hunger occurs.

One approach to controlling calorie intake is to use a Hunger/ Fullness Scale (Toolbox E). This scale can help the user know when he/she is truly hungry and should eat and when he/she feels satisfied and should stop eating. The following instructions can be used when teaching others how to use this tool:

"When you feel like you should eat, ask yourself if your body is giving you hunger signals (growling stomach, empty stomach, shakiness, light-headed, irritable, anxious) or if you are eating because you think you should (the clock says a certain time or because others are eating). Only eat when your body tells you it is time for food. After you start eating, slow down to allow your body a chance to tell you when it is full. Stop eating 2 or 3 times during each meal and ask yourself if you are still hungry or if you are feeling satisfied. When you are finished with your food, recognize your hunger/fullness number. Always try to stay between a 3 and 7 on this scale. If you let this number get too low, you are more likely to over eat once you start eating. If your number get too high, you may have consumed more calories than what you needed. Do not let your body get too hungry or too full. This may mean that you eat a small snack frequently during the day and rarely eat a large meal."

References

1. U.S. Department of Agriculture and U.S. Department of Health and Human Services. Dietary Guidelines for Americans, 2010. 7th Edition, Washington, DC: U.S. Government Printing Office. December 2010.
2. Williams MH. Nutrition for health, fitness and sport, 8th Ed. McGrawHill Companies. Boston, MA. 2007.
3. American College of Sports Medicine: Position Stand on Exercise and Fluid Replacement. Med Sci Sports Exerc 1996;28(1):i-vii.

5   Sleep

Objectives
1. List the adverse health effects of inadequate sleep.
2. Recall the recommendation for the appropriate amount of sleep for adults.
3. List strategies that can lead to more successful sleep.

Out of all the lifestyle medicine activities that are important to healthy living, one is so important that we are advised to devote a full one-third of each day doing it. This activity is, of course, sleep. Most people think of sleep as a time when our bodies and minds simply shut down and relax. On the contrary, when we sleep our bodies and minds are very active carrying out a number of vital tasks that keep us healthy and allow us to function at our best when we are awake. Sleep has a restorative quality for our bodies, and because of that, it is sometimes called "the great restorer."

In 1910, most people slept an average of 9 hours per night.[1] Today, studies have shown that most adults in America average less than 7 hours of sleep each night.[1] Like many other factors that affect lifestyle medicine activities, the current nature of our society is adversely affecting our sleep. The modern way of living in America promotes staying awake longer with 24 hours a day, 7 days a week access to entertainment, nighttime work hours, and many other activities that did not exist in 1910.[1]

The prevalence of sleep loss is significant among American adults. It is estimated that as many as 70 million Americans may be affected by chronic sleep loss or sleep disorders. More that one-third of American adults report that sleep loss adversely effects their work performance and social life at least a few days each month.[1] It is estimated that inadequate sleep costs the U.S. approximately $16 billion in direct health care expenditures and $50 billion in lost productivity each year.[1]

Not getting enough sleep has been associated with an increased prevalence of cardiovascular disease (CVD), stroke, heart disease, hypertension, diabetes, weight gain and cognitive impairment. Chronic sleep loss is also associated with an increased risk of premature death.[1] Interestingly however, the discussion in *Chapter 1, Introduction to Lifestyle Medicine* regarding lifestyle balance is exemplified with sleep in that there may also be health risks associated with sleeping too much.

✓ **Fast Fact:** People with diabetes are more likely to report sleep problems than those without diabetes.

Heathy Sleep Recommendations

One of the interesting, and largely unknown, aspects about sleep is that the amount needed by each individual to avoid daytime sleepiness can vary from person to person. Additionally, the amount of sleep needed throughout a lifespan also varies depending on age. The U.S. Department of Health and Human Services (HHS) provides recommendations on the number of sleep hours that each person should attain:[1]

•Newborns: 16-18 hours/day
•Preschool children: 11-12 hours/day
•School aged children and adolescents: at least 10 hours/night
•Teenagers: 9-10 hours/night
•Adults: 7-8 hours/night
•Older adults: 7-8 hours/night

The Physiology of Sleep

The basic sleep physiology concerning how we fall asleep involves an endogenous sleep/wake cycle that is thought to be under the primary control of two suprachiasmatic nuclei (SCN) that are located in the hypothalamus of the brain.[2] This endogenous sleep/wake cycle, sometimes referred to as circadian rhythm, is synchronized to the ambient light/dark cycle of the day.[2] Many complex factors are in play to regulate the sleep/wake cycle, however the most significant influence on the synchronization of the sleep/wake cycle appears to be environmental light received through our eyes.[2]

Another key component to the sleep/wake cycle is a hormone called melatonin.[1,2] Partially in response to signaling from the SCN, and partially in response to the onset of darkness, the pineal gland releases melatonin to promote sleep during normal periods of darkness.[2] Like the SCN, the release of melatonin is dependent upon environmental light and darkness. Brighter light suppresses melatonin release and darkness increases melatonin release.[2] Additionally, the type and wavelength of the light can have varying degrees of influence on melatonin release.[2] For example, red-wavelength light has the least effect on melatonin release, while blue-wavelength light has demonstrated the greatest effect on melatonin suppression.[2]

✓ **Fast Fact:** When healthy adults are given unlimited opportunity to sleep, they sleep on average between 8 and 8.5 hours a night.[1]

A great deal of research has been conducted on the effects of blue-wavelength light and sleep loss. Examples of blue light include fluorescent light bulbs, LED lights, television light, computer screens, smart phones and other mobile computing devices. Blue light can be beneficial during the daylight hours by increasing attentiveness, reaction time and mood.[3] However, exposure to blue light within a few hours of bedtime can adversely affect sleep.[3] More significantly, working the night shift and being exposed to light at night has been linked to breast cancer, prostate cancer, diabetes, heart disease, and obesity.[3] One study showed that shifting the circadian rhythm can increase blood sugar levels into the pre-diabetes range and can decrease the hormone leptin, making it more difficult to control appetite.[3]

Tips for decreasing exposure to blue light include:

•Avoid looking at blue light screens (computer, TV, phone) 2 to 3 hours before bedtime.
•Read with an incandescent light bulb rather than LED lights.
•If working a night shift, consider wearing blue-blocking glasses.
•Expose yourself to natural sunlight during the day.

Sleep Stages

During sleep, the brain stays active by cycling through several stages of distinctive patterns of electrical activity or brain waves.[1] There are two basic types of sleep that encompass four distinct stages of sleep. The stages of sleep repeat several times throughout the night varying in duration. The first type of sleep is called non-rapid eye movement (REM) sleep. Non-REM sleep consists of three stages:[1]

Non-REM Stage 1 (N1). Light sleep, easily awakened, muscles relaxed with occasional twitches, eye movements are slow.

Non-REM Stage 2 (N2). Eye movements stop, slower brain waves with occasional bursts of rapid brain waves.

Non-REM Stage 3 (N3). Considered the "restorative" stage that is necessary for feeling well rested and energetic during the day, deep sleep, occurs soon after falling asleep, mostly during the first half of the night, difficult to awaken, large slow brain waves (Delta waves), heart and respiratory rates are slow, muscles are relaxed.

The second type (and fourth stage) of sleep is called **REM sleep**. This stage usually occurs about 90 minutes after falling asleep, with longer and deeper periods of this stage occurring during the second half of the night.[1] During this stage of sleep, the respiratory rate, heart rate and blood pressure are irregular, the eyes move rapidly, and dreams typically occur. REM sleep stimulates the brain regions that are used to learn and make memories. Other sleep stages may do this as well.[1]

The four sleep stages repeat themselves continuously throughout the night. As the nighttime hours progress, REM sleep time becomes longer, while time spent in N3 becomes shorter.[1] Overall, almost one-half of the total sleep time is spent in N2 and about one-fifth in N3 and one-fifth in REM sleep.[1]

Sleep and Chronic Disease

Sleep (both lack of sleep and adequate amounts) has been shown to play an important role in the prevention and management of chronic diseases such as CVD, stroke, heart disease, hypertension, diabetes, obesity and cognitive impairment.[1] Below is a brief summary of the importance of sleep as is related to chronic diseases.

Cardiovascular Disease. Research has shown that during Non-REM sleep, the heart rate slows and blood pressure decreases as deeper sleep is attained. The nightly dip in blood pressure appears to be important for cardiovascular health and may to be absent when adequate sleep is not attained.[1] During REM sleep, the fluctuations in heart rate, blood pressure, and respiratory rate during dream periods are thought to promote cardiovascular health.[1] On the other hand, inadequate sleep has been shown to have adverse health effects. Research has demonstrated that a lack of sleep can increase the stress hormones epinephrine and cortisol, thereby not allowing the cardiovascular system adequate rest.[1] Additionally, inadequate sleep may trigger the production of C-reactive proteins, an inflammatory marker that may indicate an increased risk for heart disease.[1]

Diabetes, Obesity and Hormones. During sleep, a number of hormones are released that regulate the body's use of energy.[1] Sleep stages appear to be linked to blood sugar levels. Inadequate amounts of overall sleep, sleep in each stage, and sleep at the wrong times of day can disrupt the normal blood sugar levels. One study showed that women who slept less than 7 hours a night were more likely to develop diabetes over time compared with those who slept 7 to 8 hours a night. In another study, researchers found that when healthy men slept for only 4 hours a night for 6 consecutive nights, their insulin and blood sugar levels rose to pre-diabetes levels.[1] Other research has shown that compared with well rested individuals, those who are sleep deprived demonstrated a 40% reduction in blood glucose tolerance, 30% decrease in acute insulin response, 25% decrease in glucose effectiveness, and an almost 25% decrease in insulin sensitivity.[1] Each of these factors are linked to metabolic abnormalities related to diabetes.

Increasing evidence is showing that a lack of sleep puts individuals at significant risk for obesity. Research is showing that sleep is a powerful regulator of appetite, energy use and therefore, weight control.[1] During healthy sleep patterns, the body produces a hormone called leptin that acts as an appetite suppressor. Further, during healthy sleep the body suppresses the production of a hormone called grehlin, that acts as an appetite stimulant. Some studies are showing that the less people sleep, the more likely they are to be overweight or obese and prefer eating foods that are high in calories and carbohydrates. This may be due to abnormal leptin and grehlin levels.[1] One study showed that individuals who sleep an average of 5 hours a night are more likely to become obese compared to those who sleep 7 to 8 hours a night.[1]

Although not a chronic disease, the body's ability to fight off acute infections is improved with adequate sleep. During periods of healthy sleep, the body produces more cytokines, a hormone of the immune system that helps fight infections.[1] Evidence suggests that inadequate sleep can hinder the body's ability fight off infections. Additionally, research shows that a lack of sleep can reduce the body's ability to produce antibodies after having received an influenza vaccination.[1]

Cognitive impairment. A complete understanding of how sleep effects cognitive function is not fully appreciated at this time. However, much research is available to show that adequate sleep does play an important role in cognition. Recent data is showing that sleep disruptions of various kinds that occur over long periods of time are linked with accelerated cognitive decline and dementia.[4]

The short-term adverse effects of inadequate sleep have been well documented. A lack of sleep is associated with slower thinking processes, faulty decision making and more risk taking, slower reaction times, greater confusion, irritability and unhappiness.[1] Additionally, learning, memory and creativity are affected by sleep. In one study, participants needed at least 6 hours of sleep to show an improvement in learning. Additionally, those who slept 8 hours outperformed those who only slept 6 to 7 hours.[1]

Common Causes of Poor Sleep

There are many reasons why 70 million Americans are not getting adequate sleep.[1] At least 40 million of these Americans are affected by a sleep disorder.[1] The four most common sleep disorders include insomnia, sleep apnea, restless leg syndrome, and narcolepsy.[1] Individuals with signs and symptoms of sleep disorders should be encouraged to talk with their primary health care providers for solutions to improve sleep.[1,5]

Common signs and symptoms of sleep disorders are listed below. Patients should seek help if they experience any of these symptoms on three or more nights per week:[1]

•It takes more than 30 minutes to fall asleep.
•Awaken several times a night with difficulty falling back to sleep.
•Awaken too early in the morning.
•Not feeling well rested in the morning despite getting 7-8 hours of sleep.
•Feeling sleepy during the day and falling asleep within 5 minutes of laying down for a nap, or falling asleep unexpectedly or at inappropriate times.
•Bed partner reports loud snoring, gasps, choking sounds or breathing stops for short periods.
•Creeping, tingling, or crawling feelings in legs that are relieved by leg movement or massage.
•Vivid dream-like experiences when falling asleep or dozing.
•Episodes of sudden muscle weakness associated with anger, fear, or laughter.
•Feeling paralyzed upon first awakening.
•Bed partner reports frequent arm and leg jerking during night.
•Regular use of stimulants to stay awake during the day.

There are also many non-sleep disorder reasons that make sleeping difficult. Several of these sleep offenders are listed below:[1]

•*Caffeine*. Effect can very from person to person but the stimulant effect from caffeine can last up to 6-8 hours.
•*Nicotine*. Acts as a stimulant and heavy smokers may wake up too early due to nicotine withdrawal symptoms.
•*Alcohol*. Although a sedative and can induce drowsiness, it prevents deep sleep and REM sleep, allowing only lighter sleep stages.
•*Medications*. Decongestants, steroids, some antidepressants, some blood pressure medications and others have been associated with poor sleep. It is recommended to check with a pharmacists if medications are suspected.
•*Depression*. Shown to cause insomnia.
•*Psychological stress*. People who are stressed have difficulty falling asleep, staying asleep and spend less time in deep sleep and REM sleep.

•*Menstrual cycle.* Hormone shifts throughout a cycle may induce more restorative sleep but may also make it difficult to sleep depending on the phase of the cycle.

•*Menopause.* Fluctuating hormone levels can lead to insomnia and hot flashes that cause sleep disruptions.

•*Large meals.* Small amounts of food before bedtime may make is easier to fall asleep, but large quantities may make it difficult to fall asleep.

•*Vigorous exercise.* Consistent daily physical activity is associated with improved sleep, but vigorous exercise close to bedtime may make it difficult to fall asleep.

Recommendations to Improve Sleep

Several techniques can be implemented to improve sleep. A list of a few of them are provided below:

•*Consistent sleep schedule.* Keep the bedtime and wake time consistent each day of the week-even weekends-and stick to a bedtime routine.

•*Physical activity.* Thirty minutes of moderate intensity physical activity each day of the week.

•*Create a good sleep environment.* Room temperature should be cool, dark, static low volume background noise, avoid blue light from TV, computer, phone, reading light, etc.

•*Avoid caffeine, nicotine, alcohol, large meals.*

•*Avoid naps after 3:00 p.m.*

•*Relax before bedtime.* Meditation, hot bath, warm non-stimulant beverage.

•*Talk with a health care provider* - if medications are the suspected cause of poor sleep.

•*Natural sunlight.* Get at least 30 minutes of natural outside sun exposure daily.

•*Obtain a comfortable sleep surface.*

•*Don't lie in bed awake.* After 30 minutes of tossing and turning, get out of bed until sleepy.

Summary Points

• 70 million Americans may be affected by chronic sleep loss or sleep disorders at a cost of about $66 billion/year.

●Adults are recommended to get 7-8 hours of sleep/night.

• Two suprachiasmatic nuclei (SCN) located in the hypothalamus and the hormone melatonin secreted by the pineal glad play a significant role in managing the sleep/wake cycle.

●Environmental light has the most significant influence on the sleep/wake cycle.

●Sleep can be divided into 4 stages (Non-Rem Stages 1, 2, 3 and REM sleep) and they cycle repeatedly throughout the night.

●Poor sleep has been associated with CVD, diabetes, obesity and cognitive impairment.

●Poor sleep can be caused by sleep disorders and other common factors.

●Several techniques are available to improve sleep quality.

Test Your Knowledge

1. Chronic sleep loss and sleep disorders cost approximately $____ billion per year in lost productivity in America.

a. 10
b. 20
c. 30
d. 40
e. 50

2. The stage of sleep that is considered to be the "restorative" stage necessary for feeling well rested and energetic during the day is:

a. Non-REM Stage 1
b. Non-REM Stage 2
c. Non-REM Stage 3
d. REM Sleep

3. It is recommended that adults get _____ hours of sleep each night.

a. 6 to 7
b. 7 to 8
c. 9 to 10
d. 10 to 11

Practical Application Tools

Sleep Diary. In *Chapter 4, Healthy Eating*, the Practical Application Tools section presented a nutrition and physical activity diary as a means to help improve eating habits. The same can be said for a sleep diary. The purpose of a sleep diary is to increase awareness of personal sleep habits and to establish a record that can be shared with a health care provider to assist in diagnosing a sleep disorder and/or devising solutions to improve sleep. Toolbox F provides an example of a sleep diary.

References

1. U.S. Department of Health and Human Services. Your Guide to Healthy Sleep. NIH Publication No. 06-5271. November 2005.
2. Doghramji K, Markov D. Advances in the management of shift-work disorder, Part I. Pathophysiology and health-related consequences. US Pharm. December 2011: 3-11.
3. Harvard Medical School. Blue light has a dark side. Harvard Health Letter. May 2012. Accessed on January 24, 2013. Available at: http://www.health.harvard.edu/newsletters/Harvard_ Health_Letter/ 2012/May/blue-light-has-a-dark-side.
4. Gever J. Bad sleep tied to cognitive decline. Medpage Today. July 19, 2012. Accessed on January 24, 2013. Available at: http://www.medpagetoday.com/MeetingCoverage/AAIC/33820.
5. Lenz TL, Markov D. Advances in the management of shift-work disorder, Part III. General role of the pharmacist in identification, treatment, and follow-up of patients with shift-work disorder. US Pharm. December 2011: 25-32.

6   Coping with Stress

Objectives

1. Describe the impact of stress on heart disease.
2. List the symptoms of chronic stress.
3. Describe healthy coping strategies for stress.

Stress is something that we live with everyday. Most of us think of stress from an unfavorable point of view, but positive stress exists as well - such as winning the big game, scoring well on a test, or getting a raise at work. Negative stress, however, is our inability to cope with life situations that we perceive as bad. Negative stress can have untoward health effects and perpetuate chronic diseases.

The U.S. Department of Health and Human Services (HHS) defines stress as, "the brains response to any demand."[1] Nationally renowned stress expert Brain Luke Seaward defines stress as, "the experience of a perceived threat (real or imagined) to one's mental, physical, or spiritual well-being, resulting from a series of physiological responses and adaptations."[2] Several individuals and organizations have tried to define stress, but no consensus definition currently exists. Because there is no agreement on the definition of stress, it is difficult for health care providers to measure stress.

We know that stress is real, we know that everyone experiences it to some degree on a regular basis, and we know that some people are able to cope with it better than others. A particular situation may be considered highly stressful to one individual, but perceived by another as "no big deal." Because stress is largely about a "perceived threat," we should not be quick to discount another individual's stress as insignificant and unimportant. The key to coping with stress is developing effective strategies which work on an individual level with the ability to manage all things perceived to be threatening.

> "People are disturbed not by a thing, but by their perception of a thing."
> Epictetus, 55-135 A.D.

The American Institute of Stress reports that 43% of all adults suffer adverse effects due to stress.[2,3] They further state that 80% of all primary care physician office visits are stress related complaints and disorders.[2,3] Additionally, it is now estimated that up to 85% of all diseases and illnesses may be stress related - including the chronic conditions of heart disease and cancer.[2]

Types of Stress

Acute Stress

Acute stress is the most common form of stress that we feel on a day-to-day basis.[2] By the very nature of its name, it is short-term stress and can come from a good situation, bad situation or neutral situation. An example of short-term good stress is the feeling of doing something exhilarating, such as snow skiing down a mountain. Short-term bad stress can come from being stuck in a traffic jam. An example of neutral situation stress may be public speaking.

Acute stress originates from the demands and pressure of the recent past and the demands and pressures of the near future. Acute stress most often does not have lasting negative effects, but too much can lead to physiological symptoms such as an upset stomach or a tension headache. Coping strategies for short-term stress can include short-term solutions like counting to "10" or taking a brisk walk. We will discuss coping strategies in more detail later in this chapter.

A second type of acute stress, called acute episodic stress, has also been identified. This type of stress is also short-term, but occurs frequently throughout the day. Typically an individual who experiences acute episodic stress has intensely stressful reactions to nearly everything that happens in life. Although the cause of the stress appears to be a single event, there may be an underlying chronic stress "fueling the fire." Other symptoms of acute episodic stress can include persistent mild headaches, migraine headaches, high blood pressure, an inability to manage tasks, always in a rush, and self-described nervous energy. Coping strategies for episodic acute stress may be similar to those used for chronic stress.

Chronic Stress

Although acute stress can produce unwanted consequences, chronic stress has a much greater affect on health.[2] Unlike acute stress, chronic stress can last for weeks, months or even years. Examples of chronic stress include poverty, a dysfunctional family situation, unhappy personal relationships, a poor working environment, the continuous management of a chronic disease, caring for another who is chronically ill, caring for aging parent combined with raising one's own children, loneliness, and shift work or nighttime work hours. A majority of the stress related illnesses that Americans suffer from are related to the inability to cope with chronic stress.

Chronic stress is significant because it develops when an individual feels that they cannot escape from an unhappy situation. Those suffering from chronic stress feel an unbearable and unrelenting perception that the cause of the stress will last "forever." The chronic nature of the situation leads to an eventual depletion of physical and mental resources through long-term attrition. The results are physical and mental exhaustion that then manifest as complex medical conditions. Physical and psychological signs and symptoms of chronic stress can include heart attack, stroke, cancer, suicide, violence, and nervous breakdown.[2] Because of the long-term and significant effects of chronic stress, health care providers should be continually vigilant of the signs and symptoms so their patients can receive the help that is needed to adequately cope with the offending stressors.

✓ **Fast Fact:** The post-World War II era brought high technology that made lifestyles easier but helped fuel the evolutionary paradox. Even though it is easier to survive in the modern era, we experience more stress.

Physiological Mechanism of Stress

Even though no standard definition of stress currently exists, researchers have been able to come to some consensus regarding the physiological mechanism of stress. The complex internal stress processing mechanism in the body is referred to as the hypothalamus-pituitary-adrenal system.[2] The Hypothalamic Pituitary Adrenal (HPA) axis is a major part of the neuroendocrine system. The HPA axis controls reactions to stress, but also plays an important role in regulating digestion, the immune system, and energy use. The HPA axis is sometimes referred to as the "stress circuit."

When stress occurs, the hypothalamic region of the brain releases corticotropin-releasing hormone (CRH). The CRH then stimulates the pituitary adrenal gland, releasing a hormone called adrenocorticotropin (ACTH). The ACTH then acts on the adrenal glands to produce epinephrine, norepinephrine, and cortisol. Epinephrine and norepinephrine increase heart rate, blood pressure, myocardial contractility and narrow arteries to prepare for a fight or flight response.

Cortisol is a steroid hormone that is often times referred to as a "stress hormone." Cortisol is involved in the regulation of blood pressure, the regulation of insulin release to maintain proper blood glucose levels, and is important for proper immune system functioning.[2] An excessive production of cortisol (i.e. resulting from chronic stress) is associated with immune system depression, impaired wound healing and many metabolic disorders of the HPA axis such as insulin resistance, obesity, and increased blood pressure. These metabolic disorders can then lead directly to diabetes and heart disease. It should be noted that brief periods of elevated cortisol are important for the "flight or fight" response and do not have harmful long-term consequences. However, long-term and excessive production of cortisol has detrimental effects on health.

Stress and Chronic Disease

After reading the brief section on the physiological mechanism of stress, it should be no surprise that chronic stress is associated with several health issues, including many chronic diseases. A few of the health problems that have been associated with chronic diseases include depression, anxiety, loss of appetite, increased appetite, loss of sex drive, tachycardia, hypertension, hypercholesterolemia, hypertriglyceridemia, gastrointestinal disorders, immune suppression, reproductive system suppression, malnutrition, obsessive-compulsive disorder, alcoholism, poorly controlled diabetes, and hyperthyroidism. Many of the disorders are thought to develop primarily as a result of either an over-responsive autonomic nervous system (elevated stress hormones) or a dysfunctional (suppressed) immune system. Disorders such as heart disease are then developed secondarily by the over-responsive autonomic nervous system via elevated stress hormones and other factors.

Heart Disease

Recently, a meta-analysis that included the pooled results of six different studies (N=118,696) showed that individuals who demonstrated "high" perceived stress were 27% more likely to develop coronary heart disease compared with those who demonstrate "low" perceived stress.[4] The authors of the meta-analysis relate the increased perceived stress affect to be similar to that of a 50 mg/dL increase in LDL-cholesterol (the bad cholesterol), a 2.7/1.4 mmHg increase in systolic/diastolic blood pressure, or five more cigarettes per day.[4] This study demonstrates that stress should be thought of as a significant CVD risk factor, similar to other more established CVD risk factors.

The two primary physiological mechanism links between stress and heart disease are elevated blood pressure and increased cortisol release. Chronic stress induces a cascade of autonomic nervous system events that not only lead to increased oxygen demand on the heart and vasculature, but eventual blood vessel wall damage and coronary heart disease. Heart related symptoms of chronic stress include increased heart rate, increased blood pressure, abnormal heart rhythms, chest pain and difficulty breathing. As discussed above, increased cortisol secretion contributes to both increases in blood pressure and adverse changes in insulin activity. Ineffective insulin activity in-turn adversely effects energy use, appetite, and body weight.

Stress and Unhealthy Lifestyle Behaviors

The causes of chronic stress may not be directly related to unhealthy lifestyle behavior, but some unhealthy behaviors can make it more difficult to cope with stress. On the other hand, participating in certain lifestyle behaviors can greatly improve our ability to cope with stress. The lifestyle activities that have shown to be especially important for coping with stress include exercise, sleep and healthy eating.

Exercise

The benefit of exercise in coping with stress may center around the body's ability to respond to stress. The more sedentary our body gets, the less efficient it is at responding to stress.[5] On the other hand, exercise appears to provide our body with a chance to practice dealing with stress. Exercise provides multiple physiological systems (all of which are involved in the stress response) a chance to communicate more closely than in a sedentary state. The cardiovascular, renal and muscular systems work under "controlled stress" and in coordination with each other during exercise. In addition, they are all controlled by the central and synaptic nervous system which is also communicating under controlled stress during exercise. The physiological adaptations of the repeated and controlled stress is thought to be the reason that consistent exercise has been shown to effectively help manage chronic stress.

✓ **Fast Fact:** The current energy expenditure of the average American today per unit of body mass is less than 38% of that of our Stone Age ancestors.

One specific example of the benefit of exercise in coping with stress has been shown with the hormone atrial natriuretic peptide (ANP).[6] Research has shown that ANP directly "softens" the body's stress response. ANP is produced by myocardial tissue (heart muscle) and as heart rate increases during exercise, so does the production of ANP. At the same time, exercise has been shown to relax the tension in skeletal muscles by breaking the stress feedback loop to the brain. Therefore, exercise works to decrease stress by promoting muscle relaxation andy by more effectively controlling and the body's response to stress.[6]

Sleep

Stress has been shown to be one of the main culprits associated with the inability to fall asleep and stay asleep. Additionally, decreased sleep makes it more difficult to cope of stress. Poor sleep quality and quantity combined with chronic stress can create a vicious cycle where both sleep and stress adversely affect each other. A lack of sleep is associated with increased cortisol production making it difficult to cope with stress, while stress itself alters the quality of both Non-REM and REM sleep, making it difficult to feel rested in the morning. Implementing effective stress coping strategies along with effective restorative sleep strategies are especially important when individuals are caught in this negative cycle of sleep and stress.

Healthy Eating

Healthy eating and stress are closely connected in many ways. The gastrointestinal (GI) system is acutely and chronically responsive to stress. Acute and chronic stress have been linked with illnesses such as ulcers, acid reflux, colitis, irritable bowel syndrome, and Chron's disease.[7] Stress adversely affects the GI system more than nearly any other physiological system in the body.

Much like the sleep/stress connection, the inability to manage stress creates a negative cycle of coping with food consumption and stress. In both acute and chronic stressful situations, one ill advised but common coping strategy is the consumption of unhealthy foods. Increased cortisol production from stress has been shown to increase the craving for refined sugar and flour. Refined sugar and flour (ex. sugar sweetened beverages, cookies, etc) have been shown to further induce the body's stress response.

Additionally, stress induces a feeling of not having the time or interest to prepare healthy meals - leading many to choose fast food or frozen dinners which contain little nutritional value. Consuming fast foods, prepackaged frozen dinners, foods high in refined sugar and flour, salt and caffeine can induce the body's stress response. Food containing these substances can lead to increases in epinephrine and norepinephrine, which in turn cause increased heart rate, blood pressure and metabolic activity.[7] In addition, foods high in saturated fats and refined sugar are linked to compromised immune responses.[7]

The reverse is also true. Healthy food consumption has been shown to reduce stress and reverse the harmful physiological effects of stress. Several healthy food choices that can help control stress include:[7]

•*Fresh fruits and vegetables*. Produce with vibrant colors such as blueberries, red peppers, green apples, and green leafy vegetables are especially high in bioflavonoids and antioxidants that can minimize the stress response.

•*Organic foods*. Although more expensive, stress experts recommend organic foods that do not contain the chemicals from herbicides, fungicides, pesticides, and fertilizers that add to physiological stress.

•*Water*. Preventing the body from becoming dehydrated is important for lots of reasons, not the least being holding back physiological stress. Water should be the beverage of choice for nearly everyone in nearly every situation.

•*Limit caffeine*. Caffeine is a substance that can trigger the stress response. Caffeine does not need to be eliminated completely, but moderation should be the norm. High levels of caffeine are not only prevalent in coffee, but in soda and chocolate as well.

•*Eliminate soda and sugar sweetened beverages*. The most significant source of unneeded calories in the American diet comes from soda and other sugar sweetened beverages. Refined sugars that are common in these beverages have been shown to induce the stress response and most contain caffeine as well.

•*Foods that are genetically modified*. Genetic modification of certain foods has become increasingly common in our food supply as manufacturers try to improve production, taste and color. Foods that have been genetically altered are being blamed for the recent increase in food allergies by causing our immune system to be overreactive. Immune system alterations cause physiological stress which then increases the likelihood of psychological stress. The most heavily genetically modified foods are corn, soy, and tomatoes.

•*Fresh herbs and spices*. Fresh herbs and spices contain antimicrobial properties that can kill or inhibit the growth of bacteria and, thereby reduce physiological stress.

•*Fiber*. Consuming adequate amounts of fiber each day is good for GI laxation and can reduce the risk for heart disease. Maintaining a healthy heart and GI tract can reduce physiological stress on the body. Good sources of fiber include fresh fruits and vegetables and whole grains.

•*Omega-3 oils*. People who consume adequate amounts of omega-3 fatty acids have demonstrated lower levels of inflammation in the body. Omega-3 oils can only be obtained from external sources such as soybean, canola and flaxseed oil, walnuts, and salmon.
•*Eat in moderation*. Excess body weight has been shown to be a major source of physiological and psychological stress.

Symptoms of Stress

The symptoms of stress can be complex and sometime difficult to identify or correlate with acute and chronic stress situations. Symptoms can vary from person to person and likewise vary from a single symptom to multiple symptoms. The following is a list of stress symptoms:

Physical symptoms
•Upset stomach, difficulty sleeping, headache, backache, constipation, diarrhea, tight chest or throat, exhaustion, accidents and injuries, craving sweet foods

Mental symptoms
•Difficulty concentrating, difficulty making decisions, forgetfulness, scary thoughts, making errors, repetitive thoughts

Emotional symptoms
•Grumpy, tense, impatient, feeling hopeless, hostile, easily upset, unable to experience pleasure from activities that were once pleasurable, lonely, depressed, anxious

Behavioral symptoms
•Excessive drinking, overeating, under eating, driving too fast, drug use, getting into arguments, becoming a loner, working too much, excessive criticism of others

Healthy vs. Unhealthy Coping

Because stress can sometimes be difficult to manage, we tend to try to make ourselves feel better through other actions or coping behaviors. Some coping behaviors can be healthy and stress reducing, while others can unhealthy and can lead to even more stress down the road.

Examples of healthy coping behaviors include: regular and consistent physical activity, adequate sleep - but not too much (7-9 hours/night), talking with a friend or family member, meditation techniques, getting involved in activities that support the community, taking time for down-time – even if it is just a few minutes, reading a book, journaling your feelings, making extra time for hobbies, listening to music, finding humor in the situation, and reflecting on the source of the stress and reframing the situation to look at it in the bigger picture of life.

Examples of unhealthy coping behaviors include: overeating, under eating, mindless TV watching, shouting at people who are not involved in the situation, violent acts, drinking alcohol, smoking, using illicit drugs, sleeping in excess, isolating from people for long periods of time, and avoiding professional help when it is needed.

Recognizing the symptoms of chronic stress is a good first step towards stress relief. A reflection activity may be helpful for some in order to identify positive and negative coping behaviors. One such activity that can be done following an acutely stressful event involves thinking about what behaviors were acted out immediately after the event. Were these behaviors positive or negative coping behaviors? Self-awareness can be a powerful tool to help manage stress.

Effective Long-Term Coping Strategies

Several years ago, it became popular for many people to have a "stress ball" to squeeze for 60 seconds when they felt excessively stressed. Although squeezing a ball contains some degree of physical activity, it is safe to safe to say that a 60 second "squeeze" may not be the most effective strategy when dealing with complex stress issues. Identifying the source of the stress is a good first step. Developing realistic strategies that can minimize the offending stress should be the next step. Some causes of stress, however, are unavoidable and maybe even unmodifiable. For these stressors, effective coping strategies are needed.

Here are four strategies for effective long-term stress relief:

1. **Set limits with technology devices.** Instant communication has become a way of life and many people think they cannot live without checking their phone, email, social network site, and TV many times each day and night. Allowing the freedom from constantly feeling the need to be connected and to disengage from technology can be a liberating and stress relieving.

2. **Meditation.** Our world is full of sensory overload that makes our brains race, even without us knowing. Meditation can quiet our minds and calm our bodies. Examples can include The Relaxation Response (see description below), yoga and prayer.

3. **Be present for and with others.** Regular engagement in activities that serve others – like volunteering or doing random acts of kindness – can help us to focus on the bigger picture of life. Taking time to serve others (even very simple acts) can make us feel part of something larger and help put our own life struggles into perspective.

4. **Regular and consistent physical activity.** As discussed above, exercise is a proven method for both acute and chronic stress management along with its many other health benefits.

The Relaxation Response

In the late 1960's, Herbert Benson, MD discovered a counterbalancing mechanism to the stress response through his research at Harvard.[8] Benson found that by activating certain areas of the brain through simple meditation/relaxation techniques, he could reduce the stress response in a similar, but opposite way that stress is be stimulated in the hypothalamus area of the brain. He defined this opposite state as "The Relaxation Response." Regular elicitation of The Relaxation Response has been scientifically proven to be an effective treatment for a wide range of stress-related disorders. In fact, to the extent that any disease is caused or made worse by stress, the research completed on The Relaxation Response has shown to improve or reverse the disease.[9]

✔ **Fast Fact:** Herbert Benson's lab at Harvard where he discovered The Relaxation Response was in the same room in which Walter Cannon performed flight-or-flight experiments 50 years earlier.

The Relaxation Response is a physical state of deep rest that changes the physical and emotional responses to stress (e.g., decreases in heart rate, blood pressure, rate of breathing, and muscle tension). The following physiological changes occur when eliciting the relaxation response:[9]

•metabolism decreases
•heart rate slows
•muscles relax
•respiratory rate slows
•blood pressure decreases
•nitric oxide levels increase

Detailed information about The Relaxation Response technique can be found at The Benson-Henry Institute for Mind Body Medicine at: http://www.massgeneral.org/bhi/basics/rr.aspx.

Summary Points

●A universal definition of stress currently does not exist.
●Up to 85% of all diseases and illnesses may be stress related.
●Chronic stress has more significant health consequences compared with acute stress.
● Chronic diseases resulting from chronic stress include heart attack, stroke, and cancer.
● Many of the diseases and illnesses from stress are thought to develop primarily as a result of either an over-responsive autonomic nervous system (elevated stress hormones) or a dysfunctional (suppressed) immune system.
● The complex internal stress processing mechanism in the body is referred to as the hypothalamus-pituitary-adrenal system.
● The lifestyle activities that have shown to be especially important for coping with stress include exercise, sleep and healthy eating.
●Symptoms of stress can be physical, mental, emotional or behavioral in nature.

• Examples of healthy coping behaviors can include exercise, meditation, journaling, talking with a friend, listening to music, and many others.

•Effective long-term coping strategies can include limiting access to technology, meditation, being present for and with others, and regular physical activity.

Test Your Knowledge

1. As many as _____% of diseases may be related to stress.

a. 10
b. 15
c. 20
d. 85

2. The following healthy eating strategy is recommended to improve stress:

a. increase caffeine consumption
b. increase fruit and vegetable consumption
c. decrease omega-3 oils consumption
d. decrease water consumption

3. An unhealthy stress coping strategy is:

a. reading
b. journaling
c. exercising
d. sleeping in excess

References

1. U.S. Department of Health and Human Services, National Institutes of Health, National Institute of Mental Health. Adult Stress-Frequently Asked Questions. Available at: *www.nimh.nih.gov/health/ publications/stress/stress_factsheet_ln.pdf.* Accessed on February 6, 2013.
2. Seaward BL. *Managing Stress. Principles and Strategies for Health and Well-Being,* 7th Ed. Jones & Bartlett Learning. Burlington, MA. 2012.
3. American Institute of Stress. Available at http://www.stress.org. Accessed on February 6, 2013.
4. Richardson S, Shaffer JA, Falzon L, Krupka D, Davidson KW, Edmondson D. Meta-analysis of perceived stress and its association with incident coronary heart disease. Am J Cardiol. 2012;110(12):1711-1716.
5. American Psychological Association. Stress. Available at: http://www.apa.org/topics/stress/. Accessed on February 6, 2013.
6. Ratey JJ. *Spark. The Revolutionary New Science of Exercise and the Brain.* Little, Brown and Company. New York. 2008.
7. The Wellness Council of America. The Low Stress Diet. Keeping the Immune System Strong in the Face of Stress. An Expert Interview with Brian Luke Seaward. Available at: http://welcoa.org/ freeresources/index.php?category=8. Accessed on February 6, 2013.
8. Benson H. *The Relaxation Response.* Harper. New York. 2001 (original publication in 1975)
9. The Benson-Henry Institute for Mind Body Medicine. The Relaxation Response. Available at: http://www.massgeneral.org/bhi/basics/rr.aspx. Accessed on February 6, 2013.

7   Alcohol Consumption

Objectives
1. Define moderate alcohol consumption.
2. Explain the risks associated with alcohol consumption.
3. Summarize the observed benefits of alcohol consumption.

Alcohol consumption can be traced through history for over 10,000 years. Today, alcohol continues to be a prevalent part of our modern society. In the United States, approximately 50% of adults currently drink alcohol on a regular basis, and another 14% drink alcohol on an infrequent basis.[1] The topic of alcohol is important in lifestyle medicine because it has been shown to both improve health and cause significant health problems. The difference between the two appears to be related to quantity, drinking pattern, gender, age, and genetic factors.

✔ **Fast Fact:** About $50 billion per year is spent on alcohol in the U.S. of which 47% is beer and 40% is wine.

The most recent recommendations regarding alcohol consumption in the United States comes from the U.S. Departments of Health and Human Services and Agriculture in the *2010 Dietary Guidelines for Americans*.[1] The recommendation states that men and women should not consume more than a moderate amount of alcohol each day. For men, this means no more than 2 drinks per day and for women no more than 1 drink per day.[1] *The Dietary Guidelines* define one drink as 12 ounces of beer, 5 ounces of wine, and 1.5 ounces of 80-proof distilled spirits (hard liquor such as gin or whiskey). Each of these quantities delivers about 12 to 14 grams of alcohol.[2] It is important to note that there is no universally accepted definition for one drink of alcohol. *The Dietary Guidelines*, however, provide a standard that most in the U.S. use to define one drink.

Alcohol and Chronic Diseases (Risk vs. Benefit)

Benefits

The benefits of moderate alcohol consumption include decreased risk for cardiovascular disease, type 2 diabetes, and gallstones. Additionally, moderate amounts of alcohol may help keep cognitive function intact with age.[1,2] Although several health benefits have been observed with alcohol consumption, it is not recommended to begin drinking or drink more frequently for the potential health benefits.[1]

Studies have shown that the pattern of alcohol consumption is more important then the type of alcohol consumed. Consuming a moderate amount of alcohol consistently throughout the week has shown to be beneficial compared with consuming the same total amount on one day per week. In fact, binge drinking has consistently demonstrated harmful health outcomes and no health benefits.[1]

Genetics may play an important role in the likelihood of benefiting from moderate alcohol consumption, especially the benefits related to cardiovascular disease. Alcohol is metabolized by an enzyme called alcohol dehydrogenase.[2] One particular variant of this enzyme is called alcohol dehydrogenase type 1C or ADH1C. The ADH1C enzyme can be either slow acting or fast acting. The fast acting ADH1C quickly breaks down alcohol after it is consumed, while the slow acting ADH1C works more slowly. Each person has two copies of the gene that matches the ADH1C enzyme. Some people have two copies of the slow acting ADH1C, some people have two copies of fast acting ADH1C, and some people have one of each.[2] Research has shown that those who consume moderate amounts of alcohol and who have two copies of the slow acting gene have a lower cardiovascular risk compared with those who have two copies of the fast acting gene.[2] It may be possible that the fast acting enzyme breaks down the alcohol at a rate too fast to experience the beneficial effects.

Cardiovascular Disease

The benefits of alcohol consumption on cardiovascular related diseases is the most widely reported benefit of all chronic diseases related to alcohol. Over 100 prospective studies have demonstrated some level of benefit from consuming moderate amounts of alcohol.

In general, an inverse relationship has been shown with moderate alcohol consumption and the risk for heart attack, ischemic stroke, peripheral vascular disease, sudden cardiac death, and death from all cardiovascular causes.[2] The effect size appears to be fairly consistent across all the studies and demonstrates a 25% to 40% reduction in risk.[2] The benefits apply to both men and women, those with and without heart disease, and in older adults.[2] However, those who benefit the greatest tend to be older with preexisting risk for heart disease, like high blood cholesterol. It is unclear whether middle-aged and young adults experience a cardiovascular benefit from alcohol.

The benefits of drinking alcohol from a physiological perspective may be related to a rise in high density lipoprotein (HDL) cholesterol and in preventing blood clot formation. It is well established that HDL-cholesterol has a cardioprotective effect and studies have shown that moderate alcohol consumption raises HDL-cholesterol levels.[2] Moderate alcohol consumption has also demonstrated improvements in several mechanisms related to blood clotting such as fibrinogen, tissue type plasminogen activator, clotting factor VII, and von Willebrand factor. These changes may prevent the formation of the blood clots that lead to heart attack and ischemic stroke.[2]

It should be noted that even though there appears to be strong observational data showing the benefits of moderate alcohol consumption and cardiovascular disease, most of the data comes from observational studies, rather than prospectively randomized studies. It is possible that the benefits observed are related to other factors such as socioeconomic and employment status, mental health, and healthy lifestyle habits such as exercise, nutrition, and tobacco abstinence.[3] It is also important to remember that the apparent benefits of alcohol consumption on cardiovascular disease are offset at higher drinking levels.

Risks

The quantity and pattern of alcohol consumed, and the gender, age and genetics of each individual are all important factors that determine if alcohol will produce health benefits or health risks. Even moderate alcohol consumption has been associated with increased risk of breast cancer, violence, drowning, and injuries from falls and motor vehicle crashes.[1]

83

Alcohol consumed at greater than moderate amounts has been shown to increase the risk for heart attack, stroke, high blood pressure, obesity, depression, anxiety, several types of cancer, liver disease, impaired cognitive function, and accidents among others. In all, alcohol consumption has been reported to cause more than 60 types of diseases in addition to many types of injuries.[4] You may recall from *Chapter 1, Introduction to Lifestyle Medicine*, the Centers for Disease Control and Prevention reports that alcohol consumption is third most common lifestyle related cause of death in the U.S.[5]

✓ **Fast Fact:** Excessive alcohol consumption is responsible for more than 80,000 deaths in the U.S. each year - half of which are due to binge drinking.[1]

The Dietary Guidelines provide the following list of circumstances in which people should not drink alcohol:[1]

•Individuals who cannot restrict their drinking to moderate levels.
•Anyone younger than the legal drinking age. Besides being illegal, alcohol consumption increases the risk of drowning, car accidents, and traumatic injury, which are common causes of death in children and adolescents.
•Women who are pregnant or who may be pregnant. Drinking during pregnancy, especially in the first few months of pregnancy, may result in negative behavioral or neurological consequences in the offspring. No safe level of alcohol consumption during pregnancy has been established.
•Individuals taking prescription or over-the-counter medications that can interact with alcohol.
•Individuals with certain specific medical conditions (e.g., liver disease, hypertriglyceridemia, pancreatitis).
•Individuals who plan to drive, operate machinery, or take part in other activities that require attention, skill, or coordination or in situations where impaired judgment could cause injury or death (e.g., swimming).[1]

Breast Cancer

One of the most well studied chronic disease risks related to alcohol consumption is breast cancer. Significant evidence exists to show that alcohol consumption increases the risk for breast cancer.[2] A meta-analysis of six studies including over 320,000 women concluded that those who regularly consume two or more drinks per day increase their risk for breast cancer by 41%.[2]

The relationship between alcohol and breast cancer may be related to folate absorption. Studies have shown that alcohol blocks the absorption of folate and inactivates folate in the blood and tissues. This may be the primary reason for the increased breast cancer risk.[6,7] It appears that women who drink alcohol and also supplement their diet with at least 600 micrograms of folate, mitigate their increased risk for breast cancer.[2,6,7]

Alcohol and Other Lifestyle Medicine Activities

Alcohol has been shown to have an affect on certain lifestyle behaviors. Although alcohol may cause drowsiness and help people fall asleep, sleep studies show that the quality of sleep after consuming alcohol is adversely effected. Moderate alcohol can induce a feeling of relaxation, which may have a positive affect on stress, but excessive alcohol consumption has been linked with violent behavior. Additionally, alcohol can be a significant source of calories that provides no nutritional value. Therefore, those who choose to consume moderate alcohol on a consistent basis should allow for the extra calories so as to not gain body weight.

Bottom Line

Alcohol consumption is an important lifestyle medicine topic because its use is highly prevalent in society and it can deliver both health benefits and health risk. The decision to consume alcohol should be made individually and with careful consideration to gender, age, past health history, genetic risks and alcohol quantities and drinking patterns. Younger and middle-aged individuals may not receive health benefits from moderate alcohol consumption and may put themselves at increased health risks - the risks may outweigh the benefits. These individuals gain more benefit from regular exercise, healthy eating, and adequate sleep. On the other hand, older men and women with a history of heart disease or risk factors may benefit from moderate alcohol consumption - the benefits may outweigh the risks. In either case, it would be wise for those who drink alcohol to have a "risk/benefit" discussion with their primary care provider.

Summary Points

● *The 2010 Dietary Guidelines for Americans* recommends that adults consume no more than a moderate amount of alcohol each day.
● A moderate amount of alcohol for women and men is 1 and 2 drinks per day, respectively.
● One drink is defined as 12 ounces of beer, 5 ounces of wine, and 1.5 ounces of 80-proof distilled spirits (hard liquor such as gin or whiskey).
● A decrease in cardiovascular disease risk appears to be the greatest benefit from alcohol consumption.
● Alcohol consumption has been reported to cause more than 60 types of diseases in addition to many types of injuries.
● Women who drink more than moderate amounts of alcohol should supplement their diet with at least 600 micrograms of folate to de-crease the risk of breast cancer.

Test Your Knowledge

1. Moderate alcohol consumption is defined as "up to _____ drink(s) per day for men" and "up to _____drink(s) per day for women."

 2,1
b. 1,2
c. 1,0.5
d. 0.5,1

2. One drink is defined as _____ ounces of wine.

a. 3
b. 5
c. 8
d. 10

3. Women who consume 2 or more drinks per day should take folate _____ micrograms/day to reduce their risk of breast cancer.

a. 200
b. 400
c. 600
d. 800

References

1. U.S. Department of Agriculture and U.S. Department of Health and Human Services. Dietary Guidelines for Americans, 2010. 7th Edition, Washington, DC: U.S. Government Printing Office. December 2010.
2. Harvard School of Public Health. The Nutrition Source. Alcohol: balancing risks and benefits. Available at: http://www.hsph.harvard.edu/nutritionsource/alcohol-full-story/. Accessed on February 12, 2013.
3. Centers for Disease Control and Prevention. Alcohol and Public Health. Fact Sheets. Available at: http://www.cdc.gov/alcohol/fact-sheets/alcohol-use.htm. Accessed on February 12, 2013.
4. Goldberg IJ, Mosca L, Piano MR, Fisher EA. AHA Science Advisory: Wine and your heart: a science advisory for healthcare professionals from the Nutrition Committee, Council on Epidemiology and Prevention, and Council on Cardiovascular Nursing of the American Heart Association. Circulation. 2001;103:472-475.
5. Mokdad AH, Marks JS, Stroup DF, Gerberding JL. Actual causes of death in the United States, 2000. JAMA. 2004;291:1238-1246.
6. Baglietto L, English DR, Gertig DM, Hopper JL, Giles GG. Does dietary folate intake modify effect of alcohol consumption on breast cancer risk? Prospective cohort study. BMJ. 2005;331:807.
7. Zhang S, Hunter DJ, Hankinson SE, et al. A prospective study of folate intake and the risk of breast cancer. JAMA. 1999;281:1632-1637.

8   Smoking Cessation

Objectives
1. Recall the prevalence of smoking in the United States.
2. Explain the effects of smoking on chronic diseases.
3. Explain the steps of a brief intervention for an individual who smokes cigarettes.

Tobacco use is the #1 lifestyle related cause of death.[1] In the United States, smoking is responsible for one in five deaths each year - about 443,000 in total.[2] Worldwide, tobacco use causes more than five million annual deaths and is expected to increase to eight million per year by 2030.[2] Based on current cigarette smoking patterns, an estimated 25 million Americans who are alive today will die prematurely from smoking-related illnesses.[2]

✓ **Fast Fact:** On average, smokers die 13 to 14 years earlier than nonsmokers.[2]

The Centers for Disease Control and Prevention (CDC) reports that in 2010, 19.3% of people in America (45.3 million) were classified as a smoker.[2] Overall, men have a slightly higher prevalence rate for smoking compared with women. In 2010, 21.5% of men smoked versus 17.3% of women.[2]

The prevalence rates among various race/ethnicities, education levels and economic status shows dramatic differences among the various groups, leading to the conclusion that these factors play an important role in tobacco use. For example, over 31% of American Indians/Alaska Natives (non-Hispanic) smoke compared with 21% of whites (non-Hispanic), 20.6% of blacks (non-Hispanic), 12.5% of Hispanics, and 9.2% of Asians (non-Hispanics).

89

Additionally, the prevalence of smoking is inversely related to education level. In 2010, over 45% of adults with a GED diploma smoked compared with only 6.3% of adults with a post graduate college degree.[2] Lastly, nearly 30% of adults who live below the poverty level smoked in 2010 compared with 18% of those above the poverty level.[2]

Healthy People 2020 is a U.S. Department of Health and Human Services lead initiative to improve the health of Americans.[3] Healthy People provides science-based, ten-year national goals on a variety of health related topics. For tobacco use in particular, the Healthy People goal by the year 2020 is to reduce the overall prevalence of smoking from 19% of Americans to 12%.[3]

✓ **Fast Fact:** Including both cigarette and smokeless tobacco marketing, the tobacco companies spent $10.5 billion on marketing in 2008, or nearly $29 million each day.[2]

Smoking and Chronic Diseases

Smoking has a harmful affect on nearly every organ in the body. The most commonly reported diseases and illnesses related to smoking are in the broad categories of cardiovascular disease, cancer, respiratory disease, and reproductive disorders. Other illnesses such as low bone density, hip fractures, peptic ulcer disease, and cataracts have also demonstrated a direct linkage with smoking.[2]

Cardiovascular Disease

Cardiovascular disease remains the #1 cause of death among Americans, with tobacco use being the #1 "actual" reason for why Americans have cardiovascular disease.[1] In particular, of the deaths from cardiovascular disease where smoking is the cause, 62% is ischemic heart disease, 16% is other heart disease, and 12% is cerebrovascular disease.[2] Other cardiovascular disease related deaths due to smoking include aortic aneurysm, atherosclerosis, and other arterial diseases.[2]

✓ **Fast Fact:** Smoking triples a middle-aged man or woman's risk of dying from heart disease.[2]

The development of atherosclerosis is the basic underlying physiological cause of most cardiovascular and cerebrovascular diseases related to smoking.[4] Atherosclerosis is the process by which blood lipids are deposited on the inner layer of the arteries, followed by a fibrosis and thickening of the arterial wall, and eventually ischemia leading to a heart attack or stroke. A key line of defense to atherosclerosis within the arterial wall are the endothelial cells. Endothelial cells are the inner most cells that line the arterial wall as blood is flowing through the arteries. Smoking has been shown to greatly disrupt the endothelial cell as well as the balance of several key elements involved in atherosclerosis. These effects directly link smoking with ischemic heart disease and stroke.[4]

Smoking has also been shown to have direct effects on platelet activation and platelet adhesion, making smokers more susceptible to a heart attack or stroke.[4] Even nonsmokers who are exposed to cigarettes through secondhand smoke can experience acute increases in the platelet's ability for sticking to one another.[4] Smoking also induces a localized inflammatory response in the lungs and elevates inflammatory markers in the circulating blood, putting the smoker at increased risk for cardiovascular disease.[4] In addition, smoking induces the release of epinephrine and norepinephrine which makes the heart work harder by causing increases in heart rate, contractility, vascular tone, and blood pressure.[4]

Lastly, there is strong evidence that supports an association between smoking and adverse blood cholesterol levels.[4] A meta-analysis of 54 studies showed that smokers have higher concentrations of the bad cholesterols (low-density lipoprotein or LDL; very low-density lipoprotein or VLDL) and lower levels of the good cholesterol (high-density lipoprotein or HDL) compared with nonsmokers. Smoking may also have a negative affect on the way cholesterol is metabolized, putting smokers at greater risk for atherosclerosis.[4]

Cancer

In general, cancer is the #2 most common cause of death in America.[2] However, among the smoking related mortalities in the United States, cancer deaths outnumber cardiovascular deaths.[2] There are nearly 161,000 cancer deaths each year related to smoking compared to nearly 128,500 cardiovascular deaths.[2] Of all the cancer deaths each year that are related to smoking, 78% are trachea, lung or bronchus cancers.[2] Other cancers caused by smoking include lip, oral cavity, pharynx, esophagus, stomach, pancreas, larynx, cervix, kidney, renal, pelvis, urinary bladder, and acute myeloid leukemia.[2] Smoking remains the most common cause of cancer and of death from cancer today.[4]

Smoking is thought to cause genetic changes in the cells that eventually lead to cancer.[4] Smoking cessation greatly leads to a decreased risk for many types of cancers. However, quitting will never fully reduce cancer risk to that of a person who has never smoked.[4] Preventing individuals from smoking the first time remains a high priority.

Secondhand Smoke

Secondhand smoke is a combination of the smoke from the burning end of a cigarette, cigar or pipe and the smoke exhaled by smokers.[2] The CDC reports that secondhand smoke contains more than 7000 chemicals, 70 of which are known to cause cancer and hundreds more considered toxic.[2]

Research has determined that there is no risk-free level of exposure to secondhand smoke. In the U.S., secondhand smoke is estimated to cause 46,000 premature deaths in nonsmokers annually from heart disease.[2] Nonsmokers who are exposed to secondhand smoke at home or at work increase their risk for developing heart disease by 25% to 30% and for lung cancer by 20% to 30%.[2] Secondhand smoke causes an estimated 3,400 lung cancer deaths each year in the U.S. among nonsmokers.[2]

Secondhand smoke has been shown to cause significant health problems in children as well. Research has demonstrated that children exposed to secondhand smoke can have inadequately developed lungs, experience more bronchitis, pneumonia and ear infections, and get sick more often, in general. In addition, children exposed to secondhand smoke have a greater incidence of asthma along with more frequent and severe asthma attacks.[2] The CDC recommends that children should be protected from secondhand smoke in vehicles, restaurants and other public places, and at home.

Smoking Cessation

The CDC reports that in 2010, approximately 69% of smokers stated that they wanted to quit smoking. In that year, approximately 52% of smokers made a quit attempt.[2] The benefits of quitting are well documented and not just related to health benefits. Smoking can have positive social, emotional and financial benefits as well.

✓ **Fast Fact:** Starting in 2002, the number of former smokers now exceeds the number current smokers.[2]

The U.S. Department of Health and Human Services sponsors a tobacco cessation website at www.BeTobaccoFree.gov. Within this website is a useful timeline that demonstrates the health benefits overtime after quitting smoking.

• Within 20 minutes
  ◦ Heart rate and blood pressure drop
• Within 12 hours
  ◦ Carbon monoxide level in the blood drops to normal
• Within 3 months
  ◦ Blood circulation and lung function improves
• Within 9 months
  ◦ Coughing episodes lesson and breathing becomes easier
• After 1 year
  ◦ Heart disease risk is cut in half
• After 5 years
  ◦ Cancer risk of the mouth, throat, esophagus and bladder are cut in half
• After 10 years
  ◦ Lung cancer risk in cut in half and larynx and pancreatic cancer risk decreases
• After 15 years
  ◦ Coronary heart disease risk is the same as a nonsmoker

Smoking Cessation in Clinical Practice

In 2000, the U.S. Department of Health and Human Services published tobacco cessation clinical guidelines entitled, "Treating Tobacco Use and Dependence." The Guidelines were subsequently updated in 2008 and are available on the U.S. Surgeon General's website.[5] The guidelines recommend that health care providers regularly assess their patients for their use of tobacco. Data in the guidelines strongly indicate that the more frequently all health care providers address tobacco cessation with their patients, the more likely that are to stop using tobacco. Health care providers are recommended to have a systematic identification, assessment and treatment program or treatment referral process established in their practice setting.[5]

The CDC reports that the majority of cigarette smokers quit without using any evidence-based cessation treatment methods.[2] However, several tobacco cessation methods have demonstrated proven effectiveness. These methods include: (1) brief clinical intervention; (2) counseling (individual, group, or telephone); (3) behavioral cessation therapies; and (4) treatments for more person-to-person contact and intensity. Additionally, tobacco cessation medications have been found to be effective for some individuals and include nicotine replacement products (over the counter and prescription) and other prescription and nonprescription medications such as bupropion SR and varenicline. The combination of medication and counseling is more effective for smoking cessation than either strategy implemented alone.[2]

Brief Clinical Intervention

Brief clinical interventions can be provided by any healthcare provider but are most relevant to primary care providers such as physicians, pharmacists, physical therapists, occupational therapists, nurses, dentists, and respiratory therapists who are bound by time constraints.[5] A brief clinical intervention generally takes about 10 minutes or less to deliver advice and assistance about quitting. The guidelines state that a wide variety of providers can implement brief interventions and these techniques have evidence to show that they are effective.[5] Each time the patient or client visits the health care professional, a brief discussion should take place regarding smoking status, at minimum.[5]

This first step in treating patients who smoke and use tobacco is to identify the users. Effectively doing this important step can set the stage for a successful intervention with an individualized treatment plan.[5] Screening patients for current or former tobacco use will result in one of four answers: (1) the patient never regularly used tobacco; (2) the patient is currently using tobacco and is now willing to make a quit attempt; (3) the patient is currently using tobacco but is not willing to make a quit attempt at this time; and (4) the patient once used tobacco but has since quit.[5] One particular strategy for treating tobacco dependence for those ready to make a quit attempt is "The 5 A's for Brief Intervention" method. The "5 A's" methods includes the following five steps: ask, advise, assess, assist, and arrange.[5]

The first step is to simply "Ask" the patient if he/she is currently using or formerly used tobacco.[5] This question can be incorporated into any part of the patient visit, but should be asked at some point during each visit.

The next step is to "Advise" or strongly urge all smokers and tobacco users to quit.[5] The harmful effects of smoking should be communicated in a manner clear to the patient and in a strong, firm and supportive voice to let the patient know that it is important to quit and that you are there to help them. It is also important to personalize the conversation in a way that makes it important for the patient to quit due to their specific health conditions, family history, or affect on children and others in the household.[5]

Third, "Assess" the patient's willingness to make a quit attempt at this time.[5] This can be anytime within the next 30 days but ideally within the next two weeks. If the patient is willing to make a quit attempt at this time, provide assistance (discussed in Step 4). If the patient agrees to participate in intensive treatment, deliver such treatment or refer him/her to an intensive clinical interventionist.

The fourth step is to "Assist" or help the patient with a quit plan.[5] This can be accomplished through several strategies. Among these strategies include (1) setting a quit date (ideally within the next two weeks); (2) tell family, friends, and coworkers about quitting and request understanding and support; (3) anticipate challenges and identify barriers to the quit attempt, especially during the critical first few weeks and include nicotine withdrawal symptoms; (4) remove tobacco products from the environment and avoid smoking in places where much time is spent (e.g., work, home, car); (5) provide supplementary materials for the patient to use as a reference that is culturally/racially/educationally/age appropriate; (6) recommend appropriate counseling; and (7) recommend the use of approved pharmacotherapy, except in special circumstances.[5] Note, if resources are not available to offer tobacco cessation assistance, a referral process should be established to transfer patients to a qualified health care professional.

The fifth and final step in the brief intervention is to "Arrange" follow-up contact with the patient.[5] Follow-up appointments with patients can be done either in person or by way of telephone. The tobacco cessation guideline reports that telephone counseling has been shown to be an effective method of assisting patients in the smoking cessation process. Follow-up contact should occur soon after the quit date, preferably during the first week. A second follow-up contact is recommended within the first month and further contact should be conducted as needed. Note that follow-up should still occur even if the patient was referred to another health care provider for the tobacco cessation program.

Tobacco Cessation Resources

Several tobacco cessation resources are available to smokers and health care providers that make available education materials and tools to effectively assist with a cessation program. Many of these resources are free of charge and sponsored by government agencies.

Quitline Service

•1-800-QUIT-NOW (http://1800quitnow.cancer.gov.). A free telephone support service that can help individuals who want to stop smoking or using tobacco. Callers have access to several types of cessation information and services.

Online Tools and Education

•CDC's How to Quit
(http://www.cdc.gov/tobacco/quit_smoking/how_to_quit/index.htm).
A free online resource that offers tips for quitting and an extensive
quit smoking resource page.

•Smokefree.gov (www.smokefree.gov). A free and comprehensive
online resource offering a step-by-step quit guide, information on
finding a tobacco cessation expert, and quitting tools.

•BeTobaccoFree.gov (www.BeTobaccoFree.gov). A free and comprehensive online resource providing live online chat help, mobile
apps, a quitting guide, and information for teens.

•U.S. Surgeon General
(http://www.surgeongeneral.gov/initiatives/tobacco/index.html). Free
online resource with evidence-based reports on the hazards of tobacco use.

Tobacco Cessation Training Program

•Rx for Change: Clinician Assisted Tobacco Cessation
(http://rxforchange.ucsf.edu/). A comprehensive resource for health
care providers to receive training and tools for implementing a tobacco cessation program at any level.

Summary Points

● Tobacco use is the #1 lifestyle related cause of death.
●In 2010, 19.3% of people in America (45.3 million) were smokers
(21.5% of men; 17.3% of women).
● Smoking triples a middle-aged man or woman's risk of dying from
heart disease.
● Smoking kills more people from cancer than any other disease -
about 161,000 people/year.
●Over one-half of smokers make at least one quit attempt each year.
●The steps of a brief clinical intervention include ask, advise, assess,
assist and arrange.

Test Your Knowledge

1. The percentage of people in America who currently smoke is approximately _____%.

a. 12%
b. 19%
c. 24%
d. 32%

2. When smokers quit smoking, the risk of coronary heart disease decreases to that of a nonsmoker after _____.

a. 24 hours
b. 1 year
c. 10 years
d. 15 years

3. A tobacco cessation brief clinical intervention can be performed by any health care professional and generally takes about _____ minutes or less.

a. 5
b. 10
c. 15
d. 20

References

1. Mokdad AH, Marks JS, Stroup DF, Gerberding JL. Actual causes of death in the United States, 2000. JAMA. 2004;291:1238-1246.
2. Centers for Disease Control and Prevention. Smoking & Tobacco Use. Available at: http://www.cdc.gov/tobacco/. Accessed on February 14, 2013.
3. U.S. Department of Health and Human Services. Healthy People 2020. Available at: http://www.healthypeople.gov. Accessed on February 14, 2013.
4. U.S. Department of Health and Human Services. The health consequences of smoking. A Report of the Surgeon General. Atlanta: U.S. Department of Health and Human Services, Centers for Disease Control and Prevention, National Center for Chronic Disease Prevention and Health Promotion, Office of Smoking and Health, 2004.
5. Tobacco Use and Dependence Guideline Panel. Treating Tobacco Use and Dependence: 2008 Update. Rockville (MD): US Department of Health and Human Services; 2008 May. Available from: http://www.ncbi.nlm.nih.gov/books/NBK63952/

Section III

Chronic Diseases

9   Obesity

Objectives
1. Recall the prevalence of obesity in the United States.
2. List the personal and health care system burdens of obesity.
3. Explain lifestyle medicine treatment strategies for obesity.

Obesity is becoming one of the most common, serious and costly chronic diseases in the United States. In 2010, 35.7% of adults (78 million) and 16.9% of children (12 million) were considered obese by the Centers for Disease Control and Prevention (CDC).[1] For U.S. men, this compares with data from 2000 where 27.5% of men were obese versus 35.5% in 2010. For women in 2000, 33.4% were obese compared with 35.8% in 2010. The CDC predicts that by 2030, approximately 42% of adults in the U.S. will be obese.

The chronic disease of obesity is considered by the CDC to be an epidemic. This is based on the rapidly increasing prevalence of obesity in a relatively short time period. For example, from 1980 to 2008, obesity rates doubled for adults and tripled for children.[2] During the past several decades, obesity rates for all population groups—regardless of age, sex, race, ethnicity, socioeconomic status, education level, or geographic region—have increased markedly.[2]

Although nearly all segments of the U.S. population have been effected by the obesity epidemic, certain segments are more affected than others. Data from the National Health and Nutrition Examination Survey between 2005 and 2008 showed that 51% of non-Hispanic black women aged 20 years or older were obese, compared with 43% of Mexican Americans and 33% of whites.[2] Among females aged 2 to 19 years, 24% of non-Hispanic blacks, 19% of Mexican Americans, and 14% of whites were obese.[2] Addressing the socioeconomic disparity that exists with obesity is a significant issue to resolve to lessen the prevalence of obesity in America.

✓ **Fast Fact:** About 17.6 million children worldwide under 5 years of age are overweight.

The Burden of Obesity

The burden of obesity is significant on both the personal and health care system levels. Obesity increases the risk for cardiovascular related diseases such as coronary heart disease, stroke, heart failure, hypertension, and dyslipidemia. Obesity increases the risk for certain cancers such as breast, colon, prostate, and endometrial. Other significant diseases resulting from obesity include diabetes, depression, chronic obstructive respiratory disease, sleep disorders, and many more.[3]

The financial burden of obesity is significant for both direct and indirect costs. In 1998, the direct medical costs associated with obesity were reported to account for about 6% of the total direct medical costs in the U.S. or about $42 billion annually.[4] By 2006, obesity was responsible for about 10% of costs or about $86 billion per year.[4] The CDC now reports that obesity costs nearly $150 billion per year.[2] On a personal level, people who were obese in 2008 had medical costs that were $1,429 more than the cost for people of normal body weight. Indirect costs such as the value of lost work, higher insurance premiums and lower wages have also been linked with obesity.

Obesity can have a significant affect on mortality. Although the obesity epidemic is a relatively recent medical phenomenon, research has already shown that it shortens overall lifespan. As the prevalence of obesity continues to increase and more research is conducted, the mortality affect of obesity will become more clear. Here is what is currently known about the affect of obesity on mortality:[3]

•A 20 year old white male with a BMI of 45 kg/m^2 will lose 13 years of life.
•A 20 year old white female with a BMI of 45 kg/m^2 will lose 8 years of life.

•A 20 year old black male with a BMI of 45 kg/m^2 will lose 20 years of life.

•A 20 year old black female with a BMI of 45 kg/m^2 will lose 5 years of life.

Pathophysiology of Obesity

The *Clinical Guidelines on the Identification, Evaluation, and Treatment of Overweight and Obesity in Adults* defines obesity as having a body mass index greater than 30 kg/m^2.[3] Body mass index (BMI) uses an equation based on height and weight [(weight (kg) ÷ height (m^2)] to assess normal versus unhealthy body weight. It is one of the most widely used obesity assessments in clinical practice. According to the *Guidelines*, a normal BMI is 18.5 to 24.9 kg/m^2 and overweight is defined as 25.0 to 29.9 kg/m^2.[3] Other methods used to assess body weight include waist circumference, waist/hip circumference ratio, body fat distribution, and body fat percentage. Debate exists as to which method most accurately predicts poor health outcomes related to obesity. Using the same method repeatedly over time, however, may be more important than the method being used to ensure that body weight trends can be accurately compared over time.

The factors that contribute to the causes of the obesity are complex. They include the personal habits and choices of each individual as well as the larger societal issues. At a societal level, it is clear that health care disparities exist for certain groups that are related to poor access to healthy foods and safe neighborhoods for exercising. Additionally, it has been well documented that our current food supply and lifestyle behaviors do not match our evolutionary biology. This leads many to believe that simply living in our modern society is a significant contributor to the obesity epidemic. Regardless of the primary root culprit, the *Guidelines* state that weight gain can occur as a result of:[3]

•Excess calorie intake
•Physical inactivity
•Hypothalamic disorder
•Endocrine disorder
•Genetic disorder

Weight gain due to a hypothalamic, endocrine, or genetic disorder is rare. For the majority of Americans, obesity is a result of excess calorie intake and too little physical activity.[3] To maintain current body weight, a balance between calories that are taken in through food consumption and calories that are expended through metabolism and physical activity is required. When the body takes in more calories than it is expending, a positive caloric balance occurs and weight is gained. When the body expends more calories than it consumes through eating, a negative caloric balance occurs and weight is lost. When calories "in" match calories "out" body weight is maintained.

Lifestyle Medicine Strategies to Treat Obesity

Because obesity is a chronic disease, long-term treatment strategies should be developed to best treat the condition. It is important to note that weight loss does not indicate a "cure" for the disease. Undoubtedly, weight loss can significantly improve overall health. However, much research has shown that the weight loss phase of a weight control program is a relatively short period of time and that the key to long-term treatment is weight maintenance after weight loss has occurred.

The concept of weight control involves three separate phases that span a lifetime and that may cycle one or more times.

1. *Cessation of weight gain.* Stop gaining weight and maintain the excess weight.
2. *Weight loss.* Achieve the desired weight loss over a given period of time.
3. *Weight maintenance.* Maintain the weight that was lost over a lifetime without significant regain. This is the most important phase of weight control.

The *Guidelines* recommend an initial reduction of body weight by approximately 10% from baseline.[2] Even a modest reduction of 10% body weight has been shown to significantly decrease the severity of obesity-related risk factors. The *Guidelines* state that it is reasonable to achieve a 10% weight loss in approximately six months. The goal is to lose at least one-half pound per week but no more than two pounds per week. Gradual weight loss over an extended period of time has been shown to improve weight maintenance success.[2]

A successful weight maintenance program is defined in the *Guidelines* as a weight regain of less than 3 kg (6.6 pounds) in two years and a sustained reduction in waist circumference of at least 4 cm.[2] The key to a successful weight maintenance program is continual observation, monitoring and encouragement by one or more healthcare providers. Long-term monitoring of body weight should be viewed similarly to other chronic diseases such as diabetes and heart disease.

✓ **Fast Fact:** New evidence is showing that as little as 5% weight loss can decrease the risk for many chronic diseases.

Healthy Eating and Obesity

As discussed in *Chapter 4, Healthy Eating*, food intake can be approached in two distinct, yet connected strategies. Healthy eating consists of food quality and quantity. It may be easy to think that total calorie consumption as the only important factor when it comes to weight loss. There are plenty of examples of "diets" that only focus on quantity such as the Twinkie diet, the grapefruit diet, and the no carb diet. Each of these "diets" have proven the simple math equation discussed above to be correct. Eating less calories then needed will result in weight loss. These "diets' have also demonstrated that it is not realistic nor healthy to adhere long-term to this type of pattern of eating. If a long-term solution to chronic disease is the goal for obesity, then the quality of the food matters as much as the quantity.

One of the basic principles of weight loss involves the calorie deficit needed to lose weight. It is well accepted that a calorie deficit of 3,500 calories is equal to one pound of weight loss. This simple equation, however, is often over simplified in clinical practice. The *Guidelines* recommend that decreasing calorie intake by 500 to 1000 calories per day will result in a weight loss of about one to two pounds per week.[2] Although this may be true by the math, several variables are involved when trying to predict weight loss such as accuracy in calorie counting, physical activity level and individual metabolism, to name a few.

Advising an individual to simply eat 500 fewer calories each day may seem like sound advice, but it is often difficult for the patient to be successful with this plan. It is difficult to estimate, on a daily basis, the total number of calories consumed. Even if the count is off by a couple hundred calories, it undermines the fundamental assumption of 3500 calories equals one pound of weight loss. An alternate method may be needed. Rather than counting calories, the best (and easiest) way to assess whether an individual is eating the appropriate number of calories is to monitor body weight and adjust calorie intake (along with participation in physical activity) based on changes in body weight over time. The Hunger/Fullness Scale presented in *Chapter 4, Healthy Eating* and in Toolbox E may be a more practical and individually specific method to estimate appropriate calorie intake rather than calorie counting.

Along with being aware of the quantity of food being consumed, food quality can make a significant difference with a weight control program. Chapter 4 presents the *2010 Dietary Guidelines for Americans*.[5] Within this chapter is an summary of healthy eating strategies that can be applied to a weight control program. Of primary importance for weight control are avoiding sugar sweetened drinks, eating plenty of vegetables, fruits and whole grains, and drinking enough water.[5] Refer to Chapter 4 and the *2010 Dietary Guidelines for Americans* for healthy eating details.

Physical Activity

Physical activity through increased activities of daily living and a structured exercise program is very important for weight control. Physical activity contributes to direct calorie expenditure leading to the caloric deficit needed for weight loss. Physical activity may also play an important indirect role in weight loss by increasing metabolic rate and decreasing calorie consumption.[6] The *Obesity Guideline* reports that the most important strategy in a weight maintenance program is exercise consistency.[3]

Chapter 3, Physical Activity, reviews the *2008 Physical Activity Guidelines for Americans* and provides the information needed for a successful physical activity program that can be used for weight control.[6] Of special note, individuals with extra body weight are generally at an increased risk for orthopedic injury and should avoid high-impact activities like running until an adequate amount of weight is lost. In addition, starting a program slowly with a gradual progression of duration rather than intensity can provide a better exercise experience and lead to greater program adherence.

In Chapter 3, it was presented that the *2008 Physical Activity Guidelines for Americans* recommends that adults achieve a minimum of 150 minutes per week of moderate intensity physical activity. This recommendation is based on evidence that overall health is improved and the risk for many chronic diseases is reduced at this level of physical activity. However, the recommended amount of physical activity for weight loss is different. Both the *Physical Activity and Obesity Guidelines* recommend that a minimum of 300 minutes per week of moderate intensity physical activity is needed for successful weight loss.[3,6] This is equivalent to 60 minutes each day. It is important to note that a gradual build-up to this amount is recommended and that all 60 minutes are not required to be completed in a single bout of exercise.

Other Weight Control Strategies

Healthy eating and physical activity may be the two most important lifestyle medicine weight control strategies, but they are not alone in the fight against obesity. The focus of this chapter (and book) is on lifestyle medicine, but other strategies should not be ignored. Behavior therapy has been shown to be effective in weight control, especially when used with healthy eating and physical activity. *Chapter 2, Health Behavior Modification* offers several strategies that could be employed in a weight control program. Additionally, bariatric surgery is a popular weight loss method and is showing success for some individuals. There are also several medications and some herbal therapies that are frequently used for weight loss.

It is important for individuals who are obese to understand that body weight is one component of their overall health. Keeping all chronic diseases and aspects of a healthy lifestyle in balance is most important. Individuals who are overweight and even obese may live a high quality and healthy life if a balanced lifestyle approach is followed and proper management of all chronic diseases are addressed. See the discussion in *Chapter 3, Physical Activity* on Fitness vs. Fatness.

Summary Points

- Over 35% of U.S. adults are currently obese with 42% estimated by 2030.
- Obesity affects nearly every segment of the population and costs nearly $150 billion per year.
- Obesity is a significant risk factor for cardiovascular disease, cancer, and diabetes.
- The fundamental pathophysiology for obesity occurs due to excess calorie intake and physical inactivity.
- The 3 phases of a weight control program is the cessation of weight gain, weight loss, and weight maintenance.
- Obesity lifestyle medicine treatment strategies of healthy eating involve the management of food quantity and quality coupled with appropriate and consistent physical activity.

Test Your Knowledge

1. The percentage of U.S. adults currently considered to be obese is:

a. 22%
b. 28%
c. 32%
d. 35%

2. The amount of accumulated moderate intensity physical activity recommend per week for weight loss is:

a. 100 minutes
b. 150 minutes
c. 200 minutes
d. 300 minutes

3. Of the three phases of a weight control program, _____ is considered to be the most important.

a. cessation of weight gain
b. weight loss
(c.) weight maintenance

References

1. Ogden CL, Carroll MD, Kit BK, Flegal KM. Prevalence of obesity in the United States, 2009–2010. NCHS data brief, no 82. Hyattsville, MD: National Center for Health Statistics. 2012.

2. Centers for Disease Control and Prevention. Chronic Disease Prevention and Health Promotion. Obesity. Halting the Epidemic and Making Health Easier At a Glance 2011. Available at: http://www.cdc.gov/chronicdisease/resources/publications/AAG/obesity.htm. Accessed on: February 19, 2013.

3. National Institutes of Health and National Heart, Lung, and Blood Institute. Clinical Guidelines of the Identification, Evaluation, and Treatment of Overweight and Obesity in Adults Executive Summary. NIH Pub. No 98-4083. 1998.

4. Finkelstein EA, Trogdon JG, Cohen JW, Dietz W. Annual medical spending attributable to obesity: payer- and service-specific estimates. Health Aff (Millwood). 2009; 28:w822–31.

5. U.S. Department of Agriculture and U.S. Department of Health and Human Services. Dietary Guidelines for Americans, 2010. 7th Edition, Washington, DC: U.S. Government Printing Office. December 2010.

6. Physical Activity Guidelines Advisory Committee. Physical Activity Guidelines Advisory Committee Report, 2008. Washington, DC: US. Department of Health and Human Services, 2008.

10   High Blood Pressure

Objectives
1. Recall the prevalence of high blood pressure in the United States.
2. List the personal and health care system burdens of high blood pressure.
3. Explain lifestyle medicine treatment strategies for high blood pressure.

It has been well known for years that high blood pressure (hypertension) is a chronic disease and is one of the leading causes of heart disease and stroke. Yet, it remains one of the most prevalent and under treated chronic conditions. Data from the Centers for Disease Control and Prevention (CDC) shows that in 2010, approximately one in three American adults had high blood pressure.[1] This is an increase from 1994 where one in four adults had the diagnosis.[1] The American Heart Association (AHA) predicts that between 2010 and 2030, hypertension will increase by nearly 10% and add an extra 27 million people in America with a new diagnosis.[2]

The prevalence of hypertension varies by age and race, but not necessarily by gender. The CDC reports that nearly the same percentage of men compared with women currently have hypertension (34.1% vs. 32.7%, respectively).[1] When looking at race, however, a clear discrepancy is observed. The current percentage of African American men with hypertension is 43% and for women is 45.7%, much higher than the U.S. population as a whole.[1] The prevalence of hypertension is also greatly influenced by age. The lifetime risk for hypertension is about 90% for both men and women who are non-hypertensive at age 55 and 65, respectively, and survive to age 80 and 85 years.[1]

Hypertension has been shown to be a greatly under treated condition. The CDC reports that of those with hypertension, 55.8% are uncontrolled.[1] This, however, has significantly improved since 1994, when over 77% of those with hypertension were uncontrolled.[1] Still today, nearly 1 in 3 Americans with hypertension are not even aware that they have the condition.[1]

The Burden of Hypertension

The World Health Organization reports that having a systolic blood pressure greater than 115 mmHg is the number one attributable risk for death throughout the world.[3] The CDC has shown that 69% of people who have a first heart attack, 77% of people who have a first stroke, and 74% of people with chronic heart failure have high blood pressure.[1] Additionally, the treatment guidelines for hypertension (JNC 7) states that high blood pressure is responsible for nearly one-half of heart attacks and chest pains and 62% of strokes.[4]

✓ **Fast Fact:** In 2008, high blood pressure was listed as a primary or contributing cause of death for about 348,000 Americans.

Target organ damage is a term often used to describe the effect that hypertension has on certain organs in the body. The five main organs that are most adversely affected by high blood pressure include the heart, brain, kidneys, peripheral vasculature, and eyes. The specific conditions that result within these organs include myocardial infarction, angina, left ventricular hypertrophy, heart failure, stroke, dementia, chronic kidney disease, peripheral arterial disease, and retinopathy.[1]

✓ **Fast Fact:** Starting with a systolic blood pressure of 115 mmHg and a diastolic blood pressure of 75 mmHg, the risk for cardiovascular disease doubles with every 20 and 10 mmHg increase, respectively.

The financial burden of hypertension is also significant. It is currently estimated that the direct medical costs attributable to high blood pressure totals nearly $131 billion per year in the U.S.[1] The indirect costs of lost productivity alone due to hypertension are reported to be $25 billion per year.[1]

Pathophysiology of Hypertension

The most recent practice guideline for hypertension was published in 2003 and is referred to as JNC 7 (The Seventh Report of the Joint National Committee of Prevention, Detection, Evaluation, and Treatment of High Blood Pressure).[4] Within JNC 7, hypertension is defined by having one of three criteria:

1. Systolic blood pressure of 140 mmHg or higher OR diastolic blood pressure of 90 mmHg or higher; or
2. Taking medication to treat high blood pressure; or
3. Being told at least twice by a physician or other health professional that you have hypertension.

Prehypertension is a condition where an individual's blood pressure is higher than ideal, but not yet considered to be hypertension. Prehypertension has been shown to be a strong indicator of impending hypertension.[4] It is defined as having a systolic blood pressure of 120 to 139 mmHg OR a diastolic pressure of 80 to 89 mmHg in addition to not taking antihypertensive medication and having not been told by a physician or other health professional that you have hypertension.[4] Nearly one-third of U.S. adults are considered to have prehypertension.[1]

According to JNC 7, the systolic blood pressure goal for all Americans without diabetes or renal disease is less than or equal to 140 mmHg AND less than or equal to 90 mmHg for diastolic blood pressure.[4] Patients with hypertension and diabetes or renal disease should obtain a treatment goal of less than or equal to 130/80 mmHg. Recently, the American Diabetes Association has revised their blood pressure recommendation for those with diabetes to be less than or equal to 140/80 mmHg.[5] These treatment goals correlate with a decrease in cardiovascular and other disease complications along with being clinically prudent for the given population.

Hypertension can be classified into two types: essential hypertension and secondary hypertension.[4] Essential hypertension occurs in 90% of all patients with high blood pressure and secondary hypertension makes up the remaining 10%. Secondary causes are a result of a separate medical condition in which one of the adverse effects is high blood pressure. Examples of secondary hypertension include chronic kidney disease, sleep apnea, excess alcohol, thyroid disorder, obstructive uropathy and many others. Many medications can also cause secondary hypertension such as non-steroidal anti-inflammatory drugs (NSAIDs), oral contraceptive hormones, certain decongestants, chronic steroid therapy, and many others.[4] Treating secondary hypertension includes treating the primary source causing the raise in blood pressure.

The pathophysiology for essential hypertension is largely un-known. Even though 90% of individuals with hypertension are clas-sified as essential, there is no clear identifiable cause for the condi-tion. Several physiological mechanisms are involved with the main-tenance of normal blood pressure and an alteration in any one mechanism may lead to hypertension. Because the mechanisms are interrelated, it is also likely that there is more than one cause for in-creased blood pressure in those with essential hypertension. Among the factors that have been studied include salt intake, obesity and insulin resistance, the renin-angiotensin system, the sympathetic nervous system, genetics, endothelial dysfunction, low birth weight and intrauterine nutrition, and neurovascular anomalies.[6] These factors are thought to ultimately lead to hypertension by affecting cardiac output and/or peripheral resistance.

Lifestyle Medicine Strategies to Treat Hypertension

There is a great deal of evidence to support the use of lifestyle medicine activities to treat hypertension. Listed below are several lifestyle medicine activities and their relative affect on decreasing systolic blood pressure. It is important to keep in mind that although each is listed separately to show their individual effect, research has shown that combining two or more lifestyle medicine activities will result in additive outcomes.[4]

•Healthy eating (DASH): ↓8 to 14 mmHg
•Reduce dietary sodium intake: ↓2 to 8 mmHg
•Physical activity: ↓4 to 9 mmHg with 150 min/week moderate in-tensity
•Decrease alcohol consumption to moderate amounts: ↓2 to 4 mmHg
•Stress control: ↓5 mmHg
•Smoking cessation: ↓3.5 mmHg
•Weight reduction: ↓5 to 20 mmHg per 10 kg of weight loss

Healthy Eating

Arguably, one of the best eating plans developed was published with JNC 7. The Dietary Approaches to Stop Hypertension (DASH) eating plan is well established, evidence-based and very specific.[4] Following the DASH eating plan has been shown to lower systolic blood pressure by 8 to 14 mmHg in eight weeks. In fact, even those who follow the DASH eating plan and do not have hypertension experience of systolic blood pressure decrease of about 7 mmHg.[4] The emphasis of the DASH eating plan is on the consumption of fruits and vegetables to increase fiber, potassium, magnesium and calcium while lowering the consumption of saturated fat, cholesterol and sodium. Much of the *2010 Dietary Guidelines for Americans* presented in *Chapter 4, Healthy Eating* is based on the DASH eating plan.[7] Refer to Chapter 4 for more details.

Reduce Sodium Intake

Although reducing sodium is part of healthy eating, it is listed separately due to the strong evidence of its affect on lowering blood pressure and recent attention that it is receiving in the literature, media and public health arenas. Research within the DASH eating plan shows that lowering dietary sodium intake to 1,500 mg per day will independently lower blood pressure regardless of other dietary changes. The systolic blood pressure lowering effects is reported to be 2 to 8 mmHg.

The current recommendation from the *Dietary Guidelines* regarding salt intake says that individuals without hypertension should not consume more than 2,300 mg per day. However, no more than 1,500 mg per day is recommended for those with a diagnosis of hypertension, have diabetes or chronic kidney disease, are African American, or in those 51 years of age and older.[4]

✔ **Fast Fact:** The average daily sodium intake for Americans age 2 years and older is 3,400 mg of which 77% comes from processed and restaurant foods.

Physical Activity

As discussed in *Chapter 3, Physical Activity*, the recommended amount of physical activity for adults is 150 minutes per week at a moderate intensity.[8] One of the reasons that the quantity of exercise is set at this level is due to its affect on lowering blood pressure. Several studies have shown that exercising will decrease total peripheral resistance in the blood vessels and subsequently lower systolic blood pressure by 4 to 9 mmHg.[8] Refer to Chapter 3 for further information regarding physical activity and exercise.

Moderate Alcohol Consumption

It is well known that excessive alcohol consumption can increase blood pressure. Studies have shown that when those who drink more than moderate amounts of alcohol each day decrease to moderate amounts or less, they experience a systolic blood pressure decrease of 2 to 4 mmHg.[4] It is unknown if blood pressure is affected in those who only consume moderate amounts and subsequently eliminate alcohol use. *Chapter 7, Alcohol Consumption* provides further information regarding the benefits and risks associated with alcohol as well as guidelines for moderate alcohol intake.

Stress Control

Emotional stress, both acute and chronic, can raise blood pressure. Stress management techniques such as meditation, relaxation, yoga and tai chi have been shown to decrease blood pressure. On average, controlling stress can decrease systolic blood pressure by approximately 5 mmHg.[4] Refer to *Chapter 6, Stress Management* for more information on managing stress.

Smoking Cessation

Smoking is the #1 "actual" cause of death in America. This is in part due to its influence on cardiovascular disease risk. Smoking, among other things, increases blood pressure both acutely after smoking and long-term to due to blood vessel damage. Smoking cessation can lower systolic blood pressure by 3.5 mmHg.[4] The positive effects on blood pressure can be measured in a little as 20 minutes after stoping cigarette smoking.

Weight Reduction

Weight loss is not a lifestyle medicine activity per se, but more of an outcome of positive lifestyle changes.[4] Never the less, it is important to include it within this section because it has shown to significantly improve blood pressure. For each 10 kg of weight loss, a 5 to 20 mmHg decrease in systolic blood pressure can be experienced. Many individual variables are involved with weight loss and account for the wide range in blood pressure effect.

Providing individuals with hypertension the tools they need to be successful in managing their condition is important. A cartoon image of the lifestyle medicine strategies to treat hypertension is in Toolbox G as a patient education tool with the full color version available at www.LM-Rx.com. The cartoon image and website help those with hypertension understand how their medication and lifestyle medicine activities interrelate when managing high blood pressure.

Summary Points

● 1 in 3 American adults has hypertension.

● The prevalence of hypertension increases with age, African American race, diabetes, kidney disease, and unhealthy lifestyle activities.

● For most Americans, the blood pressure goal is less than 140 mmHg systolic AND less than 90 mmHg diastolic.

● Most Americans with hypertension have essential hypertension, for which there are no specific identifiable causes.

● The lifestyle medicine activities that have been shown effective at lowering blood pressure include healthy eating, reduced dietary sodium, physical activity, moderate alcohol consumption, stress control, smoking cessation, and weight loss.

● Participating in more than one lifestyle medicine activity can have an additive affect on lowering blood pressure.

Test Your Knowledge

1. Approximately ____% of Americans with hypertension do not have it adequately controlled.

a. 24
b. 37
c. 55
d. 62

2. Following the DASH eating plan can lower systolic blood pressure by _____ mmHg.

a. 2-7
b. 8-14
c. 14-17
d. 17-20

3. Participating in more than one lifestyle medicine activity can have an additive affect on lowering blood pressure.

a. True
b. False

References

1. Centers for Disease Control and Prevention. High Blood Pressure. High Blood Pressure Facts. Available at: http://www.cdc.gov/bloodpressure/facts.htm. Accessed on February 20, 2013.
2. Heidenreich PA, Trogdon JG, Khavjou OA, Butler J, Dracup K, et al. Forecasting the future of cardiovascular disease in the United States. A policy statement from the American Heart Association. Circulation. 2011;123:933-944.
3. World Health Organization. The World Health Report 2002 - Reducing Risks, Promoting Healthy Life. Available at: http://www.who.int/whr/2002/en/. Accessed on February 20, 2013.
4. Chobanian AV, Bakris GL, Black HR, Cushman WC, Green LA, Izzo JL, Jones DW, et al. Seventh report of the joint national committee on prevention, detection, evaluation, and treatment of high blood pressure. Hypertension. 2003; 42:1206-1252.

5. American Diabetes Association. New standards of care suggest less intensive blood pressure goals for people with diabetes. Available at: http://www.diabetes.org/for-media/2012/ADA-2013-SoC.html. Accessed on February 20, 2013.
6. Beevers G, Lip GY, O'Brien E. The pathophysiology of hypertension. BMJ. 2001;322:912-916.
7. U.S. Department of Agriculture and U.S. Department of Health and Human Services. Dietary Guidelines for Americans, 2010. 7th Edition, Washington, DC: U.S. Government Printing Office. December 2010.
8. Physical Activity Guidelines Advisory Committee. Physical Activity Guidelines Advisory Committee Report, 2008. Washington, DC: US. Department of Health and Human Services, 2008.

11   High Blood Cholesterol

Objectives
1. Recall the prevalence of high blood cholesterol in the United States.
2. List the personal and health care system burdens of high blood cholesterol.
3. Explain lifestyle medicine treatment strategies for high blood cholesterol.

High blood cholesterol is one of the most significant risk factors for heart disease. According to the Centers for Disease Control and Prevention (CDC), nearly 32 million Americans above the age of 20 years had a total blood cholesterol level considered to be "high" in 2012.[1] The CDC also reports that 71 million American adults (33.5%) have a LDL cholesterol ("bad" cholesterol) level considered to be too high.[1,2] Unfortunately, only one-half of American adults with high blood cholesterol receives treatment for the condition.[3] Additionally, two out of three American adults with high blood cholesterol are not treated effectively.[3]

Looking specifically at the prevalence of high LDL cholesterol (LDL-C) among men and women in America, shows that differences depend on race. More non-Hispanic white women (32%) had high LDL-C compared with men (30.5%). However, among non-Hispanic blacks more men (34.4%) had high LDL-C compared with women (27.7%). This is also the case with Mexican Americans, however the gap is even wider (41.9% of men versus 31.6% of women).[1]

Despite the high prevalence of high blood cholesterol among American adults, progress has been made over the previous decade. Since 1999, the percentage of American adults with high total cholesterol has decreased by about 5%.[1] In addition, the treatment of individuals with high LDL-C has increased from about 28% in 2002 to over 48% in 2008 (partially due to guideline revisions).[1]

> ✓ **Fast Fact:** It is thought that many people do not consider high blood cholesterol as a medical burden because most of the time there are no symptoms when levels are high.

The Burden of High Blood Cholesterol

The primary burden with high blood cholesterol is its affect on increasing cardiovascular disease risk. People with high blood cholesterol have about two times the risk for heart disease as those with a desirable level of cholesterol.[2] As stated above, about one-third of American adults have high blood cholesterol and only one-third of these individuals are managed effectively. This puts a significant number of people at increased risk for a heart attack, stroke and vascular disease. Cardiovascular disease (CVD) costs the United States an estimated $300 billion each year in direct medical expenses or about $1 of every $6 U.S. health care dollars spent.[3] Appropriately managing high blood cholesterol is an effective CVD prevention strategy.

Pathophysiology of High Blood Cholesterol

Cholesterol comes from two sources - our bodies make cholesterol and we consume it in foods. The liver and other cells make about 75% of our blood cholesterol with the remaining 25% coming from the food we eat.[4] There are two fundamental points that should be noted about cholesterol: (1) our bodies produce all the cholesterol that we physiologically require without the need to take in extra through our diet, and (2) dietary cholesterol can only come from animal sources. Understanding these two points can help to understand how lifestyle behaviors play an important role in cholesterol management.

Certain environmental, genetic and pathologic factors influence the production of cholesterol in the liver. The lifestyle behaviors of excessive alcohol consumption, cigarette smoking, a very high carbohydrate diet, and physical inactivity can all contribute to the over production of blood cholesterol. In addition, obesity and diabetes can contribute to high blood cholesterol levels. Other conditions such as hypothyroidism, chronic renal failure, and nephrotic syndrome have also been shown to lead to high cholesterol. Certain mediations such as corticosteroids, estrogens, beta-blockers, thiazide diuretics, and protease inhibitors can increase blood cholesterol as well.[2]

High blood cholesterol, sometimes called dyslipidemia, can be diagnosed based on one of several abnormal blood lipid (fat) and lipoprotein concentrations. The major blood lipids involved include:

•Triglycerides
•Cholesterol (also called lipoproteins)
        ◦High-density lipoprotein cholesterol (HDL-C)
        ◦Low-density lipoprotein cholesterol (LDL-C)
        ◦Very low-density lipoprotein cholesterol (VLDL-C)
        ◦Chylomicrons
•Phospholipids

Triglycerides are a type of blood lipid. The body makes triglycerides from the unused calories that result from overeating and are stored in fat cells. Hormones then release triglycerides for energy between meals. When excess calories are consumed on a regular basis, high triglyceride levels (called hypertriglyceridemia) can be measured. Hypertriglyceridemia is an independent risk factor for heart disease.

Elevated lipoprotein concentrations (except HDL-C) have been shown to be atherogenic or lead to atherosclerotic disease. Atherosclerosis is the process by which lipids are deposited on the inner layer of arteries, resulting in fibrosis and thickening of the arterial walls. This process can then lead to a heart attack or stroke. Low density lipoprotein cholesterol is a major cholesterol transport lipoprotein that has been directly correlated with heart disease risk. High density lipoprotein cholesterol, on the other hand, performs reverse cholesterol transport by taking excess cholesterol from tissues, such as coronary arteries, to be metabolized.

The most recent clinical guidelines for the management of high blood cholesterol was initially published in 2002, with an subsequent update published in 2004.[2] The guidelines are called, *The Third Report of the Expert Panel on Detection, Evaluation, and Treatment of High Blood Cholesterol in Adults (ATP III)*.[2] The recommended levels for the primary cholesterol components in ATP III are as follows:

•Total cholesterol - less than 200 mg/dL
•LDL cholesterol - dependent upon risk factors (less than 160 or 130 or 100 or 70 mg/dL)
•HDL cholesterol - 40 mg/dL or higher (60 mg/dL or higher is preferable)
•Triglycerides - less than 150 mg/dL

As of spring 2013, a revision of the blood cholesterol guidelines (ATP IV) has yet to be published. It is anticipated that the updated guidelines will be released in late 2013. It is likely that the cholesterol recommendations listed above will change in ATP IV and will be published on the National Heart, Lung and Blood Institute's (NHLBI) website for health care professionals at: http://www.nhlbi.nih.gov/health/indexpro.htm. The reader is encouraged to check the NHLBI website for the updated guidelines.

✓ **Fast Fact:** It is recommended that adults 20 years and older have their blood cholesterol checked every 3 to 5 years and more often if risk factors are present.

Lifestyle Medicine Strategies to Treat High Blood Cholesterol

Participating in lifestyle medicine activities is important for the treatment of high blood cholesterol, primarily due to their effects on decreasing CVD risk, in general. There is a great deal of evidence to show that specific lifestyle medicine activities will independently decrease one or more cholesterol components. Listed below are several lifestyle medicine activities and their relative effect on specific blood cholesterol components. It is important to keep in mind that although each is listed separately to show their individual effect, research has shown that combining two or more lifestyle medicine activities will result in additive outcomes. Within the APT III guidelines, the lifestyle medicine activities are referred to Therapeutic Lifestyle Changes or TLC.[2] As with the ATP III guidelines, the newly released guidelines are also expected to emphasize lifestyle activities as an important part of cholesterol management.

•Decrease saturated fat intake: LDL-C ↓8% to 10%
•Decrease dietary cholesterol intake: LDL-C ↓3% to 5%
•Increase soluble fiber intake: LDL-C ↓3% to 5%
•Supplement dietary plant sterols/stanols: LDL-C ↓5% to 15%
•Physical activity: triglycerides ↓28%; HDL-C ↑7%
•Moderate alcohol consumption: may ↑HDL-C; LDL-C ↓5% (when decreased from heavy consumption)
•Smoking cessation: smoking increases LDL-C, total cholesterol, triglycerides, and decreases HDL-C
•Weight loss: LDL-C ↓5% to 8%

Healthy Eating

When looking at the list above, it is easy to see that many of the lifestyle medicine activities that have been shown through research to lower LDL-C are dietary related. The ATP III guidelines state that following the dietary recommendations listed in the guidelines will result in a LDL-C lowering of 20% to 30%.[2] Approximately 25% of blood cholesterol levels are a result of dietary intake.

Studies have shown that every 1% increase in the consumption of calories from saturated fat correlates with a 2% increase in LDL-C.[2] The opposite has also shown to be true. For every 1% decrease in the consumption of saturated fat calories, a 2% decrease in LDL-C can be attained.[2] Decreasing saturated fat intake to less than 7% of total calories per day can decrease LDL-C by 8% to 10%. A few of the primary sources of saturated fat include beef, poultry, butter, cream, cheese, whole milk, coconut oil, palm oil, and cocoa butter.

Decreasing dietary cholesterol intake to less than 200 mg per day can decrease LDL-C by 3% to 5%. Dietary cholesterol can only be derived from animal sources. The primary sources of dietary cholesterol in the American diet include meat (especially organ meat), poultry, seafood (especially shrimp and crayfish), diary products, and egg yolks.

Increasing dietary fiber, in general, has been shown to prevent chronic diseases such as heart disease and diabetes. All dietary fibers are found naturally in the plants we eat. However, not all fibers are created equally. All dietary fibers are either soluble or insoluble. Soluble fibers attract water and form a gel, which results in slowing down digestion. This can help lower blood cholesterol levels by inhibiting the absorption of dietary cholesterol. In addition, the slowed food absorption can help more adequately control insulin levels. Consuming soluble fiber can also make you feel full by delaying food from being emptied from your stomach - helping control body weight. Sources of soluble fiber include oatmeal, oat cereal, oat bran, lentils, beans, flaxseed, nuts, apples, oranges, strawberries, blueberries, cucumbers, celery, and carrots.

Insoluble fiber does not dissolve in water so it passes through the gastrointestinal (GI) track quickly and intact. By doing so, insoluble fiber also allows food and waste to pass through the GI track more quickly and helps prevent constipation. Insoluble fibers are mostly found in whole grains and vegetables such as whole wheat, wheat bran, brown rice, bulgar, celery, broccoli, cabbage, tomatoes, carrots, dark leafy vegetables, and raisins.

The *2010 Dietary Guidelines for Americans* recommends that total daily intake of dietary fiber should be 14 grams per 1000 calories consumed.[5] For women, this is approximately 25 grams per day and for men this is about 38 grams per day. In the TLC portion of the ATP III guidelines, it is recommended to consume at least 5 to 10 grams of soluble fiber each day to help reduce LDL-C by 3 to 5%.[2]

Plant stanols and sterols are also recommended in ATP III to individuals with high blood cholesterol to reduce LDL-C.[2] Studies have shown that plant-derived stanols/sterol esters at dosages of 2 to 3 grams per day lower LDL-C levels by 6% to 15% with a maximum LDL lowering effect occurring with 2 grams per day.[2] Dietary consumption of plant stanols/sterols can be obtained from commercially available products containing plant sterols/stanols (i.e. spreads, juices, tablet formulation, and others).

Physical Activity

Physical activity, especially purposeful exercise, is a critical piece of the treatment plan for individuals with high blood cholesterol. The purpose of exercising for these individuals is primarily to lower the risk for CVD, diabetes and to control body weight. Studies have shown that exercise can greatly effect triglycerides by lowering blood levels nearly 30% with at least 150 minutes of moderate intensity activity per week.[2,6] In addition, regular exercise may be the single best method to date for boosting HDL-C. Interestingly, however, exercise does not have a significant affect on total or LDL cholesterol levels. It is important to remind those with high blood cholesterol, however, that the purpose of exercising for the treatment of high blood cholesterol it to decrease the risk for heart disease - the same purpose as taking medications to control cholesterol. Following the *2008 Physical Activity Guidelines for Americans* is the best exercise recommendations for those with high blood cholesterol.[6] Refer to *Chapter 3, Physical Activity* for more detailed information.

Moderate Alcohol Consumption

Compared with healthy eating and physical activity, data is limited on the affect of alcohol consumption and cholesterol. It is known that heavy alcohol consumption can be a cause for high total and LDL cholesterol and triglyceride levels. Studies have shown that decreasing alcohol consumption to moderate levels can lower LDL-C by about 5%. Additionally, in *Chapter 7, Alcohol Consumption* is a discussion about the positive affect that moderate alcohol consumption can have on HDL-C. One of the theories why moderate alcohol consumption appears to lower heart disease risk is the boost that it may be giving to HDL-C. More research in the area is needed, however, before confidently "prescribing" moderate alcohol consumption to decrease heart disease risk. Refer to Chapter 7 for more detailed information.

Smoking Cessation

As discussed in detail in *Chapter 8, Smoking Cessation*, smoking and tobacco use has the most significant negative influence on CVD risk compared to all other lifestyle behaviors. Specific to cholesterol, smoking has been shown to increase LDL-C by 1.7%, total cholesterol by 3%, triglycerides by 9.1%, and decrease HDL-C by 5.7%.[2] Smoking cessation is justifiable for many reasons, not the least being its direct effect on cholesterol. Refer to *Chapter 8* for more detailed information.

Weight Loss

Weight loss is not a lifestyle medicine activity per se, but more of an outcome of positive lifestyle changes. Nevertheless, it is important to include it within this section because it has shown to significantly improve blood cholesterol levels. A weight loss of 10 pounds has been shown to lower LDL-C levels by 5% to 8%, independent of the effects of healthy eating and physical activity.[2] Refer to *Chapter 9, Obesity* for more detailed information regarding weight loss.

Providing individuals with high blood cholesterol the tools they need to be successful in managing their condition is important. A cartoon image of the lifestyle medicine strategies to treat high blood cholesterol is in Toolbox H as a patient education tool with the full color version available at www.LM-Rx.com. The cartoon image and website help those with high blood cholesterol understand how their medication and lifestyle medicine activities interrelate when managing high blood cholesterol.

Summary Points

• Nearly 32 million Americans above the age of 20 years had a total blood cholesterol level considered to be "high" in 2012.

• The primary burden with high blood cholesterol is its affect on increasing cardiovascular disease risk.

• The liver and other cells make about 75% of blood cholesterol with the remaining 25% coming from food.

• The lifestyle behaviors of excessive alcohol consumption, cigarette smoking, a very high carbohydrate diet, and physical inactivity can all contribute to the over production of blood cholesterol.

•Healthy eating, physical activity, smoking cessation, moderate alcohol consumption, and weight loss have all shown to have a positive affect on blood cholesterol management.

Test Your Knowledge

1. It is estimated that individuals with high blood cholesterol who adhere to the dietary recommendations discussed in the ATP III guidelines can experience a _____% reduction in LDL-C.

a. 5 to 10
b. 10 to 20
c. 20 to 30
d. 30 to 40

2. For every 1% decrease in the consumption of saturated fat calories, a ___% decrease in LDL-C can be attained.

a. 0.5
b. 1
c. 2
d. 3

3. Soluble fiber has been shown to lower LDL-C levels by _____%.

a. 1 to 2%
b. 3 to 5%
c. 5 to 8%
d. 9 to 11%

References

1. Centers for Disease Control and Prevention. Cholesterol. Statistical Reports. Available at: http://www.cdc.gov/cholesterol/ statistical_reports.htm. Accessed on February 26, 2013.
2. National Institutes of Health, National Heart, Lung, and Blood Institute. Third report of the national cholesterol education program (NCEP) expert panel on Detection, evaluation, and treatment of high blood cholesterol in adults (Adult Treatment Panel III). NIH Publication No. 02-5215. September 2002.
3. Centers for Disease Control and Prevention. CDC Newsroom. Press Release. Most American with High blood pressure and high cholesterol at unnecessary risk for heart attack and stroke. Available at: http://www.cdc.gov/media/releases/2011/p0201_vitalsigns.html. Accessed on February 26, 2013.
4. American Heart Association. About Cholesterol. Available at: http://www.heart.org/HEARTORG/Conditions/ Cholesterol/ AboutCholesterol/About-Cholesterol _UCM_001220_Article.jsp. Accessed on February 26, 2013.
5. U.S. Department of Agriculture and U.S. Department of Health and Human Services. Dietary Guidelines for Americans, 2010. 7th Edition, Washington, DC: U.S. Government Printing Office. December 2010.
6. Physical Activity Guidelines Advisory Committee. Physical Activity Guidelines Advisory Committee Report, 2008. Washington, DC: US. Department of Health and Human Services, 2008.

12   Diabetes

Objectives
1. Recall the prevalence of diabetes in the United States.
2. List the personal and health care system burdens of diabetes.
3. Explain lifestyle medicine treatment strategies for diabetes.

Diabetes in one of the most debilitating chronic diseases in America. In 2010, diabetes affected 25.8 million Americans, or about 8.3% of the total U.S. population.[1] Of those with diabetes, 18.8 million have a diagnosis and the remaining 7 million are undiagnosed.[1] The incidence of diabetes is higher when looking specifically at the adult population, however. The Centers for Disease Control and Prevention (CDC) reports that 11.3% of Americans over the age of 20 years have diabetes. The incidence increases to 26.9% when looking at those 65 years and older.[1]

The incidence of diabetes is nearly the same for both adult men and women. Approximately 13 million men (11.8%) over the age of 20 have diabetes compared with 12.6 million women (10.8%) in the same age group.[1] Non-Hispanic black adults have higher incidence compared with non-Hispanic white adults, 18.7% versus 10.2%, respectively.[1] Among American Indians and Alaska Natives, however, the overall incidence is estimated at 16.1%, but is as high 33.5% in certain American Indian populations.[1]

The Centers for Disease Control and Prevention (CDC) predicts that by the year 2050, as many as 1 in 3 American adults will have diabetes. The International Diabetes Federation predicts that diabetes will increase by 54% worldwide by the year 2030.

Prediabetes is a condition in which individuals have a blood sugar level higher than normal, but not high enough to be diagnosed with diabetes.[1] People with prediabetes have an increased risk for developing type 2 diabetes, heart disease and stroke.[1] The CDC reports that in 2008, 35% of U.S. adults (79 million Americans) had prediabetes. In addition, approximately one-half of all those 65 years and older have prediabetes.[1]

The Burden of Diabetes

The personal and health care system burden of diabetes is significant. Overall, the risk of death among people with diabetes is about twice that of people of a similar age without diabetes.[1] Based on U.S. death certificates, diabetes was the seventh leading overall cause of death in 2007.[1] It is thought, however, that deaths related to diabetes are underreported. The CDC states that only 35% to 40% of those who die and have diabetes, have diabetes listed on the death certificate.[1]

Diabetes increases the risk for several diseases and disorders. Among the most common chronic diseases affected by diabetes include heart disease and stroke, hypertension, blindness and eye problems, kidney disease, nervous system disease, depression, and dental disease. Other conditions related to diabetes include amputations, pregnancy complications, biochemical imbalances, and an increased susceptibility to pneumonia and influenza.[1]

One of the most prevalent health burdens related to diabetes is cardiovascular-related diseases. Adults with diabetes have heart disease death rates that are 2 to 4 times higher than those without diabetes.[1] The risk for stroke is also 2 to 4 times higher for those with diabetes.[1] In addition, over 65% of adults 20 years and older with a diagnosis of diabetes, have high blood pressure.[1]

✓ **Fast Fact:** At least 65% of individuals with diabetes die from causes related to the heart or blood vessels.

Concomitant debilitating and costly chronic diseases are highly prevalent in those with diabetes. About 60% to 70% of people with diabetes have mild to severe forms of nervous system damage.[1] Diabetes is the leading cause of new cases of blindness among U.S. adults and over 28% of people with diabetes aged 40 years and older have retinopathy.[1] Additionally, diabetes is the leading cause of new cases of kidney failure and about one-third of people with diabetes have severe periodontal disease.[1]

Another significant complication related to diabetes is depression. People with diabetes are twice as likely to have depression than people without diabetes.[1] It is also interesting that depression is associated with a 60% increased risk of developing type 2 diabetes. Therefore, diabetes can lead to depression and depression can lead to diabetes. It is widely known that having both depression and diabetes can significantly complicate diabetes management.

The direct and indirect costs associated with diabetes in 2007 totaled $174 billion. Of this total, $116 billion resulted from direct medical expenses with $58 billion coming from indirect expenses such as disability, work loss, and premature mortality. The CDC reports that average medical expenditures among people with diagnosed diabetes were 2.3 times higher than what expenditures would be without diabetes.[1]

✓ **Fast Fact:** Studies show that diabetes self-management education leads to reductions in costs related to care.

Pathophysiology of Diabetes

Diabetes occurs as a result of an absolute or relative lack of insulin to the cells of the body resulting in high blood glucose levels or hyperglycemia. Diabetes can be diagnosed using the hemoglobin A1C test.[2] Individuals who have an A1C of 6.5% or greater are considered to have diabetes.[2] An A1C of 5.7% to 6.4% is considered to be prediabetes. Individuals with an A1C in this range are considered to be at high risk for future diabetes, with those at 6.0% or greater at very high risk.[2]

The two most common types of diabetes are type 1 and type 2. In addition to these, women can develop diabetes as a result of the stress during pregnancy and is referred to as gestational diabetes. Other, less common types of diabetes can be caused by infections, drugs, genetic defects, pancreatic destruction, and endocrinopathies. We will keep our focus on the treatment of type 1 and type 2 diabetes.

Type 1 diabetes occurs in 5% to 10% of those with diabetes and is characterized by an absolute lack of insulin or the inability of the pancreas to make and secrete insulin.[2] This inability to produce insulin results from an autoimmune destruction of the beta cells of the pancreas. Most people with type 1 diabetes are diagnosed before age 30 years, with peak diagnosis between the ages of 12 and 14 years. Family history of type 1 diabetes is not significant and the primary focus of treatment involves insulin. Those with type 1 diabetes are at an increased risk for CVD and other conditions and therefore, exercise and healthy eating activities are important from a lifestyle medicine perspective.

Type 2 diabetes accounts for 90% to 95% of those with diabetes. It is characterized by a relative lack of insulin due to insulin resistance at the tissue level, a defect in insulin secretion, or an increase in hepatic glucose output. As type 2 diabetes progresses, all three of these pathophysiological processes may be happening at the same time.

Type 2 diabetes is most frequently diagnosed at ages older than 40 years. Unfortunately, there is a trend towards an increasing incidence of type 2 diabetes before the age of 40 years. Unlike type 1 diabetes, the risk for type 2 diabetes is strongly linked to genetics and family history. Obesity and physical inactivity are thought to be primary contributors to type 2 diabetes along with advancing age, family history, and race. Therefore, the treatment of type 2 diabetes is heavily focused on lifestyle medicine activities such as exercising, healthy eating and weight loss, in addition to oral antidiabetic agents. Insulin may also be needed in some individuals as type 2 diabetes progresses.

Lifestyle Medicine Strategies to Treat Diabetes

Participating in lifestyle medicine activities is very important for the treatment of both type 1 and type 2 diabetes. As stated above, the primary purpose for those with type 1 diabetes is CVD risk management. For type 2 diabetes, however, there is a great deal of evidence to show that specific lifestyle medicine activities will independently contribute to the management of blood glucose levels along with decreasing CVD risk. Listed below are several lifestyle medicine activities and their relative affect on blood sugar management. It is important to keep in mind that although each is listed separately to show their individual effect, research has shown that combining two or more lifestyle medicine activities will result in additive outcomes.

•Decrease total carbohydrate intake: A1C ↓3.5%
•Exercise (aerobic): A1C ↓0.64%
•Exercise (resistance training): A1C ↓0.67%
•Weight loss: A1C ↓0.7% with 5% to 10% weight loss
•Smoking cessation: 25 or more cigarettes per day doubles risk for type 2 diabetes
•Alcohol consumption: moderate amounts are associated with lower A1C

✓ **Fast Fact:** The Diabetes Prevention Program was one of the first programs to demonstrate that lifestyle medicine activities could significantly reduce the risk of developing diabetes.

Healthy Eating

The American Diabetes Association (ADA) has concluded that for both type 1 and type 2 diabetes, the total amount of carbohydrate consumed each day is more important than the type of carbohydrate consumed to adequately control blood glucose. However, the best mix of carbohydrate, protein and fat calories appears to vary depending on individual circumstances. It is highly recommended that individuals with diabetes consult with a dietitian or other diabetes nutrition expert to design an individualized healthy eating plan.[2] An individualized plan will depend on metabolic status (lipid profile, renal function) and/or food preferences.[2] The ADA states it is likely that several different types of eating plans may be effective in managing diabetes, including Mediterranean-style, plant-based, low-fat, and low-carbohydrate.[2] One particular study has shown that lowering carbohydrate intake to about 30% of total calories in people with poorly controlled type 2 diabetes, can decrease A1C by 3.5% over a 6 month time period.[4] This is equivalent to an estimated average glucose (eAG) of about 100 mg/dL.

Physical Activity

Two different types of exercises have shown to be effective at managing blood glucose levels: aerobic and resistance training. Following an aerobic exercise program such as recommended in *Chapter 3, Physical Activity* has been shown to lower A1C by 0.64% (eAG of -19 mg/dL).[5] Likewise, a resistance training program of 3 sets of 13 repetitions, on 10 exercises, performed 2 to 3 times per week has shown a similar 0.67% A1C decrease (eAG of -18 mg/dL).[5]

The positive affects that exercise has on blood glucose control is a result of an insulin-like affect that takes place due to repeated muscle contractions. Both aerobic and resistance training activities have shown to enhance the uptake of glucose allowing for better glycemic control, even in the presence of glucose deficiencies.[2] Physical activity also improves glucose tolerance, improves insulin sensitivity, and decreases insulin requirements. Muscular blood glucose uptake not only occurs during exercise, but remains elevated for several hours post exercise. The effects of a single bout of aerobic exercise on improving the action of insulin and blood glucose tolerance can be observed for up to 72 hours post exercise. For this reason and others, the ADA recommends that those with type 2 diabetes exercise at least three days per week with no more than two consecutive days between bouts of exercise.[2]

There are several safety precautions for exercising with diabetes that should be mentioned. Individuals with diabetes should be aware of their blood glucose levels before and after a bout of exercise to maintain proper blood glucose control and to prevent injury and complications. It is recommended to avoid exercise if fasting glucose is greater than 250 mg/dL and ketosis is present and to use caution if blood glucose is greater than 300 mg/dL and no ketosis is present.[2] Another important factor for those taking insulin before exercising is to consider the injection site with the type of exercise being performed. Studies have shown that injecting insulin directly into an area of the body that is about to be exercised can alter the absorption of the insulin and, therefore, alter the glycemic control. For example, injecting insulin into the thigh just prior to cycling has shown an increased rate of insulin absorption during the first 10 minutes of activity by 135% and by 50% over the entire exercising time (60 minutes) compared to rest.[6] This increased absorption may result in a greater decrease in blood glucose during the recovery period following exercise compared with injecting insulin into the abdomen. The ADA recommends avoiding insulin injections into exercising limbs to lower the risk of hypoglycemia associated with exercise. The preferred injection site is in the abdomen.[2]

Weight Loss

Weight management is fundamental to the management of diabetes and blood glucose levels. Just as increasing body weight can lead to insulin resistance, losing body weight can reverse this process and allow for better blood glucose control. It has been shown in one study that losing an average of 8.6% body weight can lead to a 0.7% decrease in A1C.[7] This correlates to an eAG of -20 mg/dL. Losing weight with both exercise and healthy eating is the most effective method to manage blood glucose and its complications for those with type 2 diabetes. Refer to Chapters 3, 4, and 9 on Physical Activity, Healthy Eating, and Obesity, respectively for more detailed information.

Smoking Cessation

As discussed in detail in *Chapter 8, Smoking Cessation*, smoking and tobacco use has the most significant negative influence on CVD risk compared to all other lifestyle behaviors. Specific to diabetes, one study showed that men who smoke 25 or more cigarettes per day were 1.94 times more likely to develop type 2 diabetes. It is uncertain if there is a direct cause and effect relationship or if the increased risk related to other unhealthy behaviors. Nevertheless, smoking cessation should be a high priority for anyone who smokes to decrease CVD risk.

Alcohol Consumption

Alcohol consumption can be a precarious activity for people with diabetes. Consuming alcohol within a short period of time, without food, and in excessive amounts can significantly affect blood glucose levels. Alcohol can have both a hypoglycemic and hyperglycemic affect making is difficult to appropriately manage blood sugar levels. However, those who consume moderate amounts of alcohol with food have shown no acute effects on blood glucose or insulin levels and one particular study showed that moderate consumption is associated with lower A1C levels compared with nondrinkers.[8] The ADA's recommendations concerning alcohol consumption for those with diabetes are the same as the recommendations for those without diabetes. These recommendations are consistent with those in the *2010 Dietary Guidelines for Americans* and listed in *Chapter 7, Alcohol Consumption.*

Providing individuals with diabetes the tools they need to be successful in managing their condition is important. A cartoon image of the lifestyle medicine strategies to treat diabetes is in Toolbox I as a patient education tool with the full color version available at www.LM-Rx.com. The cartoon image and website help those with diabetes understand how their medication and lifestyle medicine activities interrelate when managing diabetes.

Summary Points

- Nearly 12% of U.S. adult have diabetes.
- The CDC predicts that by 2050, one-third of Americans will have diabetes.
- The risk of death among people with diabetes is about twice that of people of a similar age without diabetes.
- Type 2 diabetes accounts for 90% to 95% of those with diabetes.
- Obesity and physical inactivity are thought to be primary contributors to type 2 diabetes.
- Lifestyle medicine activities such as healthy eating, exercising and weight loss can significantly improve blood glucose control.
- Exercise has an insulin-like effect to help control blood glucose.

Test Your Knowledge

1. A hemoglobin A1C of _____% or greater is diagnostic for diabetes.

a. 5.5
b. 5.7
c. 6.5
d. 7.0

2. Both aerobic exercise and resistance training have been shown to decrease A1C levels.

a. True
b. False

3. The ADA recommends that those with type 2 diabetes exercise at least three days per week with no more than _____ consecutive day(s) between bouts of exercise.

a. 1
b. 2
c. 3
d. 4

References

1. Centers for Disease Control and Prevention. Diabetes Public Health Resource. 2011 National Diabetes Fact Sheet. Available at: http://www.cdc.gov/diabetes/pubs/estimates11.htm#1. Accessed on February 27, 2013.

2. American Diabetes Association. Standards of Medical Care in Diabetes - 2012. *Diabetes Care January 2012 vol. 35 no. Supplement 1 S11-S63.*

3. Centers for Disease Control and Prevention. Diabetes Public Health Resource. Basics About Diabetes. Available at: http://www.cdc.gov/diabetes/consumer/learn.htm. Accessed on February 27, 2013.

4. Haimoto H, Sasakebe T, Wakai K, Umegaki H. Effects of a low-carbohydrate diet on glycemic control in outpatients with severe type 2 diabetes. Nutr Metab. 2009;6:1-5.

5. Boule NG, Haddad E, Kenny GP, Wells GA, Sigal RJ. Effects of exercise on glycemic control and body mass index in type 2 diabetes mellitus: a meta-analysis of controlled clinical trials. JAMA. 2001;286:1218-1227.

6. Lenz TL, Lenz NJ, Faulkner MA. Potential interactions between exercise and drug therapy. Sports Med. 2004;34:293-306.

7. The Look AHEAD Research Group. Reduction in weight and cardiovascular disease risk factors in individuals with type 2 diabetes. Diabetes Care. 2007;30:1374-1383.

8. Ahmed AT, Karter AJ, Warton EM, Doan JU, Weisner CM. The relationship between alcohol consumption and glycemic control among patients with diabetes: The Kaiser Permanente Northern California Diabetes Registry. J Gen Intern Med. 2008;23:275-282.

13   Coronary Artery Disease

Objectives

1. Recall the prevalence of coronary artery disease in the United States.
2. List the personal and health care system burdens of coronary artery disease.
3. Explain lifestyle medicine treatment strategies for coronary artery disease.

The most common type of heart disease in the United States is coronary artery disease (CAD), also called coronary heart disease (CHD).[1] Coronary artery disease is defined by the U.S. National Library of Medicine as a narrowing of the small blood vessels that supply blood and oxygen to the heart.[2] The most common outcome of CAD is angina, but the most significant outcome for CAD is a heart attack.[1] Risk factors for CAD include smoking, physical inactivity, unhealthy eating, stress, poor sleep, over consumption of alcohol, obesity, high blood pressure, high blood cholesterol, and diabetes.

The most recent data from the American Heart Association (AHA) shows that 15.4 million Americans (6.4%) over the age of 20 years have CAD.[3] The prevalence is higher in men compared with women, 7.9% versus 5.1%, respectively. It is estimated that in 2013, approximately 635,000 Americans will be hospitalized or die of a new coronary attack and an additional 280,000 will have a recurrent attack. The average age of a first heart attack for men is 64.7 years and for women is 72.2 years. The lifetime risk for developing CAD after the age of 40 years is 49% for men and 32% for women.[3]

✓ **Fast Fact:** Every day in America, an adult will have a heart attack every 44 seconds.

The incidence of CAD varies by race and gender. The incidence for CAD among non-Hispanic white men is 8.2% and for women is 4.6%.[3] For non-Hispanic blacks, however, the incidence is higher in women than men, 7.1% versus 6.8%, respectively. Among Mexican Americans, CAD is prevalent in 6.7% of men and 5.3% of women.[3] The prevalence of CAD is lowest among Asians where it estimated to be only 4.3% overall.[3]

The Burden of Coronary Artery Disease

Coronary Artery Disease ranks as the number one cause of the death among American adults. One out of every six deaths in America is due to CAD.[3] The American Heart Association estimates that about 15% of those who experience a heart attack will die from the event and 80% of the people who die are 65 years of age and older. The AHA also states that, on average, 16.6 years of life are lost because of a heart attack.[3]

✔ **Fast Fact:** 50% of men and 64% of women who die suddenly from a heart attack have no previous symptoms of CAD.

The cost burden of CAD is significant. In 2009, it is estimated that the direct and indirect costs of CAD were $195.2 billion.[3] In 2006, the hospital costs for a heart attack were reported to be $14,009 per discharge. For ischemic heart disease, the average discharge was reported to be $10,630 per person.[3]

It is estimated that between the years 2013 and 2030 the medical costs of CAD will increase by 100%.[3] During this time period the indirect costs associated with cardiovascular disease are expected to increase by 53%, with CAD accounting for the largest portion of this increase (43%).[3]

Each year the American Heart Association publishes an update on *Heart Disease and Stroke Statistics.* [4] The 2012 Update provided a very succinct list of cardiovascular disease risk (CVD) factor statistics. They are as follows:

Top Ten Things To Know about the AHA Heart and Stroke Statistics - 2012 Update:[4]

1. From 1998 to 2008, cardiovascular disease (CVD) death rates declined 30.6%. However, CVD is still the leading cause of death in the U.S. Declines in stroke death rates now rank stroke as the 4th leading cause of death.

2. From 2007 to 2008, the cost of CVD increased by over $11 billion.

3. Hypertension - An estimated 76.4 million U.S. adults ≥20 years of age are hypertensive.

4. Cholesterol - An estimated 98.8 million adults ≥20 years of age have total serum cholesterol levels ≥200 mg/ dL; 33.5 million have total serum cholesterol levels ≥240 mg/ dL.

5. Diabetes - An estimated 18.3 million Americans ≥20 years of age have physician-diagnosed diabetes. An additional 7.1 million adults have undiagnosed diabetes, and about 81.5 million adults have pre-diabetes.

6. Physical Activity - Only 20.7% of adults meet the federal guidelines for physical activity. Among 9th through 12th graders, only 37.0% meet the recommendations.

7. Healthy Diet – Less than 1% of U.S. adults meet the definition for a ideal healthy diet; essentially no children meet the goal.

8. Smoking - 19.8% of boys and 19.1% of girls in grades 9-12 report being current smokers. Among adults, 21.2% of men and 17.5% of women over age 18 years are smokers.

9. Body Mass Index - Overall, 68% of U.S. adults are overweight or obese (72% of men and 62% of women). Thirty-two percent of children ages 2-19 are overweight or obese (32% of boys and 31% of girls).

10. When compared to previous trends for adults, there have been improvements in CVD and stroke mortality, a decreased prevalence of high cholesterol, and an increase in physical activity participation.

However, there have been relatively no changes in prevalence of hypertension and smoking, and a worsening prevalence of diabetes and obesity.

Pathophysiology of Coronary Artery Disease

Angina (suboptimal blood flow) and heart attack (complete lack of blood flow in certain arteries) occurs as a result of atherosclerosis.[5] Atherosclerosis is a localized accumulation of blood fat (lipid) and fibrous tissue within the arteries. This process can occur in the heart and in other arteries that affect the brain (ischemic stroke) and lower extremities (peripheral arterial disease). Atherosclerosis involves the production of fatty streaks in the coronary arteries that eventually lead to a fibrous plaque formation in the vessel.[5] If atherosclerotic plaque grows to the point of occluding greater than 50% of the arterial lumen, anginal symptoms (shortness of breath, chest discomfort) can occur with and without physical activity as more of the arterial lumen is taken up by the plaque. When 95% or greater of the arterial lumen is occupied by plaque, coronary blood flow is functionally absent and results in a heart attack.[5]

Most heart attacks, however, occur as a result of an atherothrombosis.[5] Atherothrombosis occurs when the fibrous plaque ruptures. During this process the lipid core of the plaque leaks out into the arterial lumen causing a thrombosis to form which can quickly break away from the site of the rupture. The thrombus then travels in the coronary vessel until it gets lodged due to the narrowing of the coronary vessels. This then inhibits blood flow to the heart tissue that is behind the thrombus causing a heart attack. The formation of atherosclerotic plaque can begin very early in life, but does not usually present itself with symptoms and CAD until adults are middle aged or older.[5]

Lifestyle Medicine Strategies to Treat Coronary Artery Disease

Each chapter reviewed in this book has discussed the effects of various topics on the risk for developing CAD or CVD, in general. Each of the lifestyle medicine activities (physical activity, healthy eating, sleep, stress management, alcohol consumption, and smoking cessation) has demonstrated that it can have a significant influence on the development and treatment of CAD. Of special importance to note for those diagnosed with CAD is the intensity of the lifestyle medicine treatment. Much has been written in the respective lifestyle medicine guidelines about the intensity of therapy for those with CAD versus those with the risk factors for CAD (i.e. obesity, high blood pressure, high blood cholesterol, diabetes) versus those who have yet to demonstrate risk factors. The intensity of lifestyle medicine therapy increases as risks increase. Examples can be seen with more aggressive restrictions on saturated fat and sodium intake. Also, target blood cholesterol levels are recommended to be lower in those with CAD versus those without CAD. In addition, most individuals with CAD participate in a supervised cardiac rehabilitation exercise program after a coronary event. This highly structured exercise setting uses a team approach to regain heart function to treat the underlying disease process.

When working with individuals who have CAD, it is very important to communicate with the other members of the individual's personal health care team. This should be done to ensure that it is safe to participate in lifestyle medicine activities and to optimize the treatment plan. In addition, optimal program adherence is more likely to occur with more members of the health care team encouraging positive lifestyle behaviors.

Summary Points

●Coronary artery disease occurs in about 6.4% of Americans and results in one out of every six deaths in America.
● The direct and indirect costs of CAD are over $195 billion per year.
●Coronary artery disease develops from atherosclerosis and can lead to a heart attack via atherothrombosis.
●Lifestyle medicine treatment increases in intensity for those with CAD compared with those without CAD.
●Working with other members of the heath care team is very important with CAD.

Test Your Knowledge

1. Coronary artery disease is the number one cause of death in the United States.

(a) True
b. False

2. The lifetime risk for developing CAD after the age of 40 years is ____% for men.

a. 24
b. 36
c. 42
(d) 49

3. Atherothrombosis occurs when the fibrous plaque ruptures.

(a) True
b. False

References

1. Centers for Disease Control and Prevention. Heart Disease. Available at: http://www.cdc.gov/heartdisease/. Accessed on March 4, 2013.
2. Medline Plus. U.S. National Library of Medicine. National Institutes of Health. Coronary Heart Disease. Available at: http://www.nlm.nih.gov/medlineplus/ency/article/007115.htm. Accessed on March 4, 2013.
3. Go AS, Mozaffarian D, Veronique LR, et al. AHA Statistical Update. Heart Disease and Stroke Statistics - 2013 Update. A Report from the American Heart Association. Circulation. 2013;127:e6-e245.
4. Roger VL, et al; on behalf of the American Heart Association Statistics Committee and Stroke Statistics Subcommittee. Heart disease and stroke statistics—2012 update: a report from the American Heart Association. Circulation. 2012: published online before print December 15, 2011, 10.1161/CIR.0b013e31823ac046. Available at: http://circ.ahajournals.org/lookup/doi/10.1161/CIR.0b013e31823ac046
5. Chilton RJ. Pathophysiology of Coronary Heart Disease: A Brief Review. J Am Osteopath Assoc. 2004;104(9):5S-8S.

Section IV

Application of Lifestyle Medicine

14   Documenting Lifestyle Medicine

Objectives
1. List examples of lifestyle medicine vital signs that could be included in a medical chart.
2. List lifestyle medicine specific information that could be included in a medical chart.

Documenting an individual's lifestyle medicine activities is an important component of a lifestyle medicine program. Similar to other types of important medical information, lifestyle medicine specific data should be documented to provide a historical record of an individual's past lifestyle medicine experiences, track progress, and to allow other members of the health care team to be fully informed about all treatment modalities. Unfortunately, most lifestyle medicine activities are only minimally recorded in a standard medical chart, or not recorded at all.

Lifestyle Medicine Vital Signs

In a typical medical chart, a patient's vital signs such as height, weight, blood pressure, heart rate, and respiratory rate are routinely recorded. Although unconventional in current practice settings, lifestyle medicine vital signs are also important to record - especially for those with a chronic disease. Tobacco use, alcohol use, and illicit drug use are all lifestyle medicine related vital signs and may currently be found in medical records. Effective documentation of lifestyle habits, however, should go well beyond these commonly recorded vital signs.

Vital signs are used to obtain a snapshot of important information about a patient. Briefly listing several lifestyle medicine related activities, such as those listed below, can serve the same purpose as traditional vital signs and provide a complete picture of a patient's progress in managing their specific chronic disease(s):

•Physical activity and purposeful exercise
•Eating habits (e.g. fruit/vegetable, whole grain consumption)
•Sleep (quantity and quality)
•Stress level, emotional well-being, and stress reduction activities
(e.g. meditation)

Other lifestyle medicine vital signs may also include:

•Body mass index and waist circumference measurements
•Barriers to implementing lifestyle medicine activities
•Social framework at home, workplace, and in the community
•Life meaning and purpose (e.g. religious beliefs)

Charting Lifestyle Medicine

A traditional medical chart contains information about a patient
such as health history, medications, procedures, lab data, and progress notes. Additional information about a lifestyle medicine program could additionally include:

•*Lifestyle medicine program details.* This sections includes initial
baseline testing, goals and specific program details for physical activity, healthy eating, sleep success, stress management, alcohol consumption, and smoking cessation.

•*Lifestyle medicine progress note.* A traditional progress note contains Subjective, Objective, Assessment, and Plan (S.O.A.P.) information documented each time a patient visits with their health care
professional. This note could be redesigned to add lifestyle medicine
information to the S.O.A.P. format.

•*Quality of life questionnaire (QOL) data.* QOL data could be as-
sessed at baseline and on an annual basis to measure the impact of
the lifestyle medicine program on self-perceived health.

•*Patient self-reflection goals.* An important part of a lifestyle medicine program is the engagement of the participant. Goal setting exercises that are driven by the participant will help improve adherence
and build a sense of ownership through a patient-center experience.

•*Nutrition and physical activity diary records.* The medical chart could serve as a repository for nutrition and physical activity diary information. A summary of the diary information may be needed if a paper diary is used due to the amount of information that would need to be stored. If an electronic diary is used, the information could be uploaded to an electronic medical chart if possible.

•*Computer generated nutrition analysis.* Information from a nutrition diary can be uploaded into a nutrition analysis software program to provide specific dietary information such as carbohydrate, fats, protein, fiber, sodium intake and more.

•*Lifestyle journal data.* A lifestyle journal can be used to track daily lifestyle related habits. Like a nutrition and physical activity diary, the information can be summarized or stored electronically in an electronic medical record.

Paper and Electronic Charting

The documentation of medical information continues to move to an electronic medical record (EMR) format which brings tremendous opportunities for documenting lifestyle medicine activities - especially for those with chronic diseases. Many electronic applications (apps) available on smart phones and other mobile devices have been developed to record lifestyle medicine related data. Some of these apps are more comprehensive in nature and are referred to as personal health records (PHR). An integration of PHR data and EMR data may provide a robust document that focuses on lifestyle medicine activities for the treatment of chronic diseases. If such a document were available where all members of a lifestyle medicine team and the patient had access, communication and overall care for chronic diseases may improve.

Summary Points

•Documenting a patient's lifestyle medicine activities is an important component of a lifestyle medicine program.
•Lifestyle medicine vital signs are important to record in a medical chart, especially for those with chronic diseases.

●Lifestyle medicine vital signs can include data such as physical activity, eating habits, sleep quantity and quality, and stress level.

●Customizing a medical chart for lifestyle medicine can include changes to the S.O.A.P. note, participant reflection goals, and nutrition analysis data.

● An integration of PHR data and EMR data may provide a robust document that focuses on lifestyle medicine activities for the treatment of chronic diseases.

Test Your Knowledge

1. Lifestyle medicine vital signs can provide a more complete picture of a patient's progress in managing their chronic condition.

a. True
b. False

2. Patient self-reflection goals is an important component to document in a lifestyle medicine program.

a. True
b. False

3. An integration of PHR data and EMR data may provide a robust document that focuses on lifestyle medicine activities for the treatment of chronic diseases.

a. True
b. False

15   Tools for Lifestyle Medicine

Objectives
1. Describe the purpose of developing a lifestyle medicine toolbox.
2. List several different examples of tools that can be used in lifestyle medicine.

When a contractor builds a house, several different types of tools are used for the different phases of the job and to adapt to the uniqueness of the house. Similarly, a lifestyle medicine program has many different phases and each individual participant is unique unto him/herself. Developing a set of lifestyle medicine tools that work with the practice setting and that are diverse and adaptable to all individuals for whom a program is being designed, is key. A lifestyle medicine toolbox is a central component to the application of the lifestyle medicine concepts discussed in this book.

The purpose of developing a lifestyle medicine toolbox is to heighten motivation, increase self-awareness, decrease barriers, improve education, and track progress. A health care provider's lifestyle medicine toolbox should be specific to his/her practice setting. The number of tools in the toolbox will depend on the patients participating in the program, the program's budget, the physical space where the program takes place, and personal preferences of the health care provider.

The bottom-line when choosing lifestyle medicine tools is to pick the one(s) that will work for an individual patient. Not every tool will work for every person and most tools will need a trial period to see if they are effective. Listed below are several examples of lifestyle medicine tools.

Program Adherence Tools

Lifestyle Journal. A lifestyle journal can be used to increase self-awareness and track progress in areas such as medication adherence, physical activity, fruit and vegetable intake, sleep, stress, alcohol intake and many others. It can also be used to record and track blood pressure, blood glucose, body weight and other personal health data. *LM Tool A* provides an example of a lifestyle journal.

Nutrition & Physical Activity Diary. Documenting food consumption in a diary format can help some people visualize their intake on a per meal, per day, or per week basis. People often times do not realize the amount of food they have eaten or the frequency to which they are eating until they see it on paper. The same can be done for physical activity. *LM Tool D* provides an example of a nutrition and physical activity diary.

Medication Pill Box. Although not a lifestyle medicine activity, medication adherence is critical for those with a chronic disease. Due to the high number of medications that some people take, it may be difficult to track adherence unless they use a pill box. Medication pill boxes have been used for years by patients as a way to organize their medications and ensure adherence.

Self-Monitoring Devices

Home Blood Pressure Monitor. Evidence has shown that patients who monitor their blood pressure at home have greater blood pressure control.[1] The devices lead to increased self-awareness and give health care providers average measurements over time that may even be more accurate than office blood pressures if "white coat hypertension" is an issue.

Blood Glucose Monitor. Crucial to the treatment plan for diabetes is the frequent measurements of blood glucose. These devices not only ensures that medications are dosed appropriately, but they provide important information about food intake and the effects of exercise on blood glucose.

Pedometer. A study published in 2007 demonstrated that individuals who wear pedometers are associated with significant increases in physical activity and decreases in body mass index and blood pressure.[2] Pedometers are an effective lifestyle medicine tool because they increase motivation, self-awareness, and provide a mechanism for people to directly monitor a personalized goal, thus leading to greater self-efficacy.[2]

Goal Setting Tools

Questionnaires to assess readiness and confidence to participate in lifestyle medicine activities. Questionnaires can be developed that list various lifestyle medicine activities where participants can rate their readiness and confidence to participate in these activities using the Transtheoretical Model of Behavior Change.[3] This information can be used to identify which lifestyle medicine activities to tackle first based on the individual's interests and motivation. An example of questionnaires such as this can be found in *LM Tool C* and a description with further details on how to use these questionnaires can be found in *Chapter 2, Behavior Modification.*

Education Tools

Online Education. Many organizations are available for patients online that provide both information about various chronic diseases and lifestyle medicine activities. Many sites are culturally sensitive and written in easy to understand language. Providing a list of credible online resources is an inexpensive way to keep people educated.

Demonstration devices. Dietitians often use props to help them educate people about proper eating habits. Examples of these can include portion control plates, bowls and cups. They can also include a comparison of serving sizes of certain foods with common nonfood items (e.g. 3 oz. of meat = size of a deck of cards; a cup of salad = size of a baseball). Educational demonstration devices can also include showing a patient with diabetes how to properly use a glucometer, a home blood pressure monitor, or pedometer. Using a visual aids to teach people with chronic disease can be very effective.

Video presentations to deliver "just-in-time" demonstrations. Offering videos about lifestyle medicine activities can be a very effective method of education. For some patients it may be the preferred method of communication over written materials.

Culturally specific materials. It is critical that the individuals receiving the educational materials can culturally relate to the information. People are more likely to engage in and change lifestyle behaviors if they perceive that what they are reading applies directly to them.

Risk Assessment Tools

Both electronic and paper-based tools are available to predict a individual's unique risk for developing cancer, osteoporosis, depression, cardiovascular disease, and others. Using these tools in a lifestyle medicine program can help motivate people to change behaviors as well as educate them about the seriousness of specific chronic conditions. These tools can be effective to show how changing certain lab values (e.g. blood pressure) can lower heart attack risk, thereby providing specific goals that the individual can more easily understand. The Framingham Heart Study, started in 1948 by the National Heart Lung and Blood Institute, has 14 risk score profiles related to cardiovascular disease. The Framingham Risk Score Profiles are scientifically valid and widely used tools that are free of charge. They can be accessed at: http://www.framinghamheartstudy.org/.

Electronic Communication Tools

Personal Health Record. Our ever changing world of enhanced technology and communication devices can help improve adherence to a health behavior change program as well as overall patient care. Implementing electronic medical records (EMR) and personal health records (PHR) into practice is becoming a standard but may also play an important role in lifestyle medicine. Individuals can use a PHR to document lifestyle activities which may also be viewed by their healthcare providers to aid in tracking progress, addressing implementation and/or adherence barriers, as well as hold the patient accountable for their lifestyle behaviors. It is predicted that this aspect of health care will, in general, continue to advance and become more widely used. It will allow for better communications between patients and their health care providers and between health care providers themselves. Specifically for lifestyle medicine, program adherence may improve as providers and patients are more closely connected.

Mobile Device Applications

The increased use of mobile devices such as smart phones, tablet computers, surface computers and others bring tremendous utility for a lifestyle medicine program. Mobile "apps" can be integrated into a lifestyle medicine program to track adherence and progress, self-monitor personal health data, set goals, educate, assess chronic disease risk, and to improve communication. Having a list of quality lifestyle medicine related "apps" may be very helpful for participants who like to use this type of technology.

Summary Points

• The purpose of developing a lifestyle medicine toolbox is to heighten motivation, increase self-awareness, decrease barriers, improve education, and track progress.
• A health care provider's lifestyle medicine toolbox should be specific to their practice setting.
• The bottom-line when choosing lifestyle medicine tools is to pick the one(s) that will work for each individual.
•Examples of lifestyle medicine tools can range from those that improve adherence and track progress, to those that educate, assess risk and improve communication.

Test Your Knowledge

1. A lifestyle medicine toolbox is a central component to the application of lifestyle medicine.

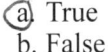 True
b. False

2. A lifestyle journal can increase an patient's self-awareness about their lifestyle habits.

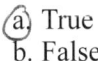 True
b. False

3. Mobile device applications have no future in lifestyle medicine.

a. True
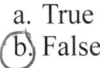 False

References

1. Pickering TG, Houston-Miller N, Ogedegbe G, et al. Call to Action on Use and Reimbursement for Home Blood Pressure Monitoring: A Joint Scientific Statement From the American Heart Association, American Society of Hypertension, and Preventive Cardiovascular Nurses Association. Hypertension. 2008; 52: 10 - 29.
2. Bravata DM, Smith-Spangler C, Sundaram V, et al. Using pedometers to increase physical activity and health. A systematic review. JAMA. 2007;298:2296-2304.
3. Prochaska JO, Johnson S, Lee P. The Transtheoretical Model of Behavior Change. In: The Handbook of Health Behavior Change, 3rd Ed. Shumaker SA, Ockene JK, Riekert KA, Editors. New York: Springer. 2009:59-83.

Section V

Lifestyle Medicine Toolbox

LM Tool A
Lifestyle Journal

The lifestyle journal is a log book that provides the user with a means of tracking day-to-day lifestyle related activities. Here is an example of what a lifestyle journal could look like:

Activity	Sun	Mon	Tue	Wed	Thu	Fri	Sat
Purposeful exercise (min)							
Fruit servings							
Vegetable servings							
Sleep (hrs)							
Alcoholic drinks							
Blood pressure							
Blood glucose							

LM Tool B
Composite Lifestyle Index

Directions: For each of the six components below, find the score that matches with how you have been doing on that particular healthy lifestyle activity over the past 2 weeks. You can calculate your *Composite Lifestyle Index (CLI)* before starting a purposeful lifestyle modification program or at any time. Record your current score and use it as a mark of comparison for a later time. Set your initial goal to be at least 20 total points. However, regardless of your score, try to increase your total points by 5 points every 4 weeks. Your ultimate goal is to achieve 40+ total points and to maintain that amount for the rest of your life. If it takes 10 years or more to achieve 40+ points, it is okay. Just keep moving forward on your journey of better health by continuously earning more points. Think of CLI it is your lifestyle grade point average (GPA).

HEALTHY EATING

On the table below, find the <u>average</u> number of <u>daily</u> servings* of combined fruits and vegetables that you consumed during the previous 2 weeks.

Score	Combined fruit and vegetable servings (servings/day)
10	10
9	9
8	8
7	7
6	6
5	5
4	4
3	3
2	2
1	1
0	0

*1 serving = medium whole piece; ½ cup of fresh, frozen or canned; ¼ cup dried

PHYSICAL ACTIVITY

On the table below, find the <u>average</u> number of total <u>weekly</u> minutes of physical activity* during the previous 2 weeks.

Score	Moderate Activities[†] (minutes/week)	Vigorous Activities[‡] (minutes/week)	Combined[#] (minutes/week)
10	150+	75+	115+
9	135-149	68-74	104-114
8	120-134	60-67	92-103
7	105-119	53-59	81-91
6	90-104	45-52	69-80
5	75-89	38-44	58-68
4	60-74	30-37	46-57
3	45-59	23-29	35-45
2	30-44	15-22	23-34
1	1-29	1-14	1-22
0	0	0	0

*Physical activity can be purposeful exercise or other bodily movements that you did for at least 10 minutes at a time (e.g. walking, exercise classes, sporting activity, yard work, taking your dog for a walk)
[†]Examples include: walking, dancing, hiking, bicycling leisurely
[‡]Examples include: jogging, running, walking up stairs, bicycling 12+ mph
[#]Combination of moderate and vigorous activities (e.g. walking + jogging + cycling)

SLEEP

On the table below, find the <u>average</u> number of hours of sleep <u>per night</u> you obtained during the previous 2 weeks.

Score	Sleep (hours/night)
10	7 to 9
9	6 ½ to 7 OR 9 to 10
8	6 to 6 ½ OR 10 to 11
7	5 ½ to 6 OR 11 to 12
6	5 to 5 ½ OR 12 to 13
5	4 ½ to 5 OR 13 to 14
4	4 to 4 ½ OR 14 to 15
3	3 ½ to 4 OR 15 to 16
2	3 to 3 ½ OR 16 to 17
1	Less than 3 OR More than 17

TOBACCO USE

On the table below, record a "10" if you <u>do not</u> use tobacco (ex. smoking or smokeless tobacco) and a "0" if you currently use tobacco.

Score	Tobacco Use Score
10	Do not use tobacco
0	Currently use tobacco

ALCOHOL CONSUMPTION

On the table below, find the <u>average</u> number* of alcoholic drinks consumed <u>per day</u> when alcohol consumption has occurred during the previous 2 weeks.

Score	Men (drinks/episode day)	Women (drinks/episode day)
10	0, 1 or 2	0 or 1
9	NA	NA
8	NA	NA
7	NA	NA
6	NA	NA
5	NA	NA
4	NA	NA
3	3	2
2	4	3
1	5 or more	4 or more

*Average number is defined as the number of drinks consumed per episode rather than the average number of drinks consumed for each day of the previous 2 weeks (e.g. A man drank alcohol on 5 days out of the previous 2 weeks. Each day that he drank he averaged 2 drinks. Therefore, his average drinks/episode day = 2 and his score = 10).

STRESS

Use the scale below to estimate your <u>average daily</u> stress over the previous 2 weeks.

Looking back at my <u>overall</u> stress level throughout the day, I would say it was:

1 = Low Stress (feeling calm and in control)
2
3 = Moderate Stress
4
5 = High Stress (feeling frantic and out of control)

Score	Stress Scale Score (average/day)
10	1
9	1 to 1.4
8	1.5 to 1.9
7	2 to 2.4
6	2.5 to 2.9
5	3 to 3.4
4	3.5 to 3.9
3	4 to 4.4
2	4.5 to 4.9
1	5

COMPOSITE LIFESTYLE INDEX (CLI)

Record your score for each healthy lifestyle activity category in the boxes below. Add all scores together to obtain your CLI.

Lifestyle Activity	My Score
Healthy Eating	
Physical Activity	
Sleep	
Tobacco Use	
Alcohol Consumption	
Stress	
TOTAL	

LM Tool C
Readiness and Confidence to Participate

READINESS TO PARTICIPATE IN LIFESTYLE ACTIVITIES*

Directions: Below is a "Readiness to Participate" ranking scale. For every lifestyle activity listed under the ranking scale, place a number for your readiness to do that activity as a 1, 2, 3, 4 or 5 according to the description on the scale.

Rating	Readiness to Participate
1	I have no interest in this activity at this time
2	I am thinking about starting this activity sometime in the next few months
3	I am making a plan to start this activity sometime within the next month
4	I have been consistently participating in this activity for the past 1 week to 6 months
5	I have been consistently participating in this activity for longer than the past 6 months

Rating	Lifestyle Activities
	Take medication as directed by a doctor and/or pharmacist
	Participate in purposeful cardiovascular exercise at least 5 times per week (e.g. walking, jogging, bicycling, exercise classes)
	Get "extra" physical activity every day (e.g. taking stairs, walking pets, parking further away in the parking lot)
	Participate in sporting activity at least 1-2 times per week (e.g. golf, volleyball, basketball, tennis)
	Participate in muscle fitness exercises 2-3 times per week (e.g. resistance training with bands, gym equipment or weights)
	Eat 5 or more servings of fruits and vegetables every day
	Eat at least ½ of my grains from whole grains (e.g. bread, cereal, pasta)
	Lose or maintain body weight
	Avoid smoking or tobacco use
	Practice stress reduction techniques every day (e.g. meditation, yoga, prayer)
	Sleep 7-9 hours every night
	Receive a flu vaccination this year
	Drink no more than two alcoholic drinks per day (or abstain from drinking alcohol)
	Wear a seat belt when driving or riding in a vehicle

CONFIDENCE TO PARTICIPATE IN LIFESTYLE ACTIVITIES*

Directions: Below is a "Confidence to Participate" ranking scale. For every lifestyle activity listed under the ranking scale, place a number that represents the confidence you have to do that activity as a 1, 2 or 3 according to the description on the scale.

Rating	Confidence to Participate
1	Very confident
2	Somewhat confident
3	Not very confident

Rating	Lifestyle Activities
	Take medication as directed by a doctor and/or pharmacist
	Participate in purposeful cardiovascular exercise at least 5 times per week (e.g. walking, jogging, bicycling, exercise classes)
	Get "extra" physical activity every day (e.g. taking stairs, walking pets, parking further away in the parking lot)
	Participate in sporting activity at least 1-2 times per week (e.g. golf, volleyball, basketball, tennis)
	Participate in muscle fitness exercises 2-3 times per week (e.g. resistance training with bands, gym equipment or weights)
	Eat 5 or more servings of fruits and vegetables every day
	Eat at least ½ of my grains from whole grains (e.g. bread, cereal, pasta)
	Lose or maintain body weight
	Avoid smoking or tobacco use
	Practice stress reduction techniques every day (e.g. meditation, yoga, prayer)
	Sleep 7-9 hours every night
	Receive a flu vaccination this year
	Drink no more than two alcoholic drinks per day (or abstain from drinking alcohol)
	Wear a seat belt when driving or riding in a vehicle

*Adapted with permission from: Gillespie ND, Lenz TL. Implementation of a tool to modify behavior in a chronic disease management program. Advances in Preventive Medicine. 2011;Article 215842, 5 pages. doi:10.4061/2011/215842.

LM Tool D
Nutrition & Physical Activity Diary

Date:		
Nutrition		
Food or Drink	**Amount**	**Time of Day**

	Total pedometer reading for the day =		
Physical Activity	**Type of Activity**	**Duration (minutes)**	**Intensity (light, moderate, heavy)**

LM Tool E
Hunger/Fullness Scale

This scale will help you know when you are truly hungry and should eat and when you feel satisfied and should stop eating. When you feel like you should eat, ask yourself if your body is giving you hunger signals (growling stomach, empty stomach, shakiness, light-headed, irritable, anxious) or if you are eating because you think you should (the clock says a certain time or because others are eating). Only eat when your body tells you it is time for food.

After you start eating, slow down to allow your body a chance to tell you when it is full. Stop eating 2 or 3 times during each meal and ask yourself if you are still hungry or if you are feeling satisfied. When you are finished with your food, recognize your hunger/fullness number. Always try to stay between a 3 and 7 on this scale. Do not let your body get too hungry or too full. This may mean that you eat a small snack frequently during the day and rarely eat a large meal. This is okay and what you body actually prefers.

Rating	Hunger / Fullness Feeling
10	Uncomfortable full - "sick" feeling
9	Stuffed - uncomfortable
8	Too full - somewhat uncomfortable
7	Full - but not uncomfortable
6	Filling up - but feel like you could eat more
5	NEUTRAL - not hungry or full
4	Slightly hungry - faint signals of hunger but could still wait
3	Hungry - clear signals of hunger (growling, empty stomach)
2	Too hungry - irritable, anxious, slight headache
1	Ravenous - will eat anything in site
0	Starving - weak, light-headed, shakes, splitting headache

Source: US Department of Veterans Affairs. National Center for Health Promotion and Disease Prevention. Hunger and Fullness. N04 Version 3.0. http://www.move.va.gov.

LM Tool F
Sleep Diary

	DATE	Wednesday 1/23/2013	
AM	Time I went to bed last night	11:00 p.m.	
	Time I woke up this morning	7:00 a.m.	
	Number of hours slept last night	8	
	Number of awakenings and total time awake last night	5 times; 2 hours	
	How long I took to fall asleep last night	30 min.	
	Medications taken last night	None	
	How awake did I feel when I got up this morning: 1 = wide awake; 2 = awake but tired; 3 = sleepy	2	
PM	Number of caffeinated drinks (soda, tea, coffee) and time when I had them today	1 drink at 8:00 p.m.	
	Number of alcoholic drinks (beer, wine, liquor) and time when I had them today	2 drinks at 9:00 p.m.	
	Nap times and lengths today	3:30 p.m.; 45 min.	
	Exercise times and lengths today	None	
	How sleepy I felt during the day today: 1 = very sleepy, struggle to stay awake; 2 = somewhat tired; 3 = fairly alert; 4 = wide awake	1	
	How stressful I felt today (on a scale of 1-5): 1 = not stressful; 5 = very stressful	4	

AM: Complete in the morning

PM: Complete in the evening

Source: USDHHS. Your guide to healthy sleep. NIH Pub. No. 06-5271. 2005

LM Tool G
Lifestyle is Medicine...for the treatment of High Blood Pressure

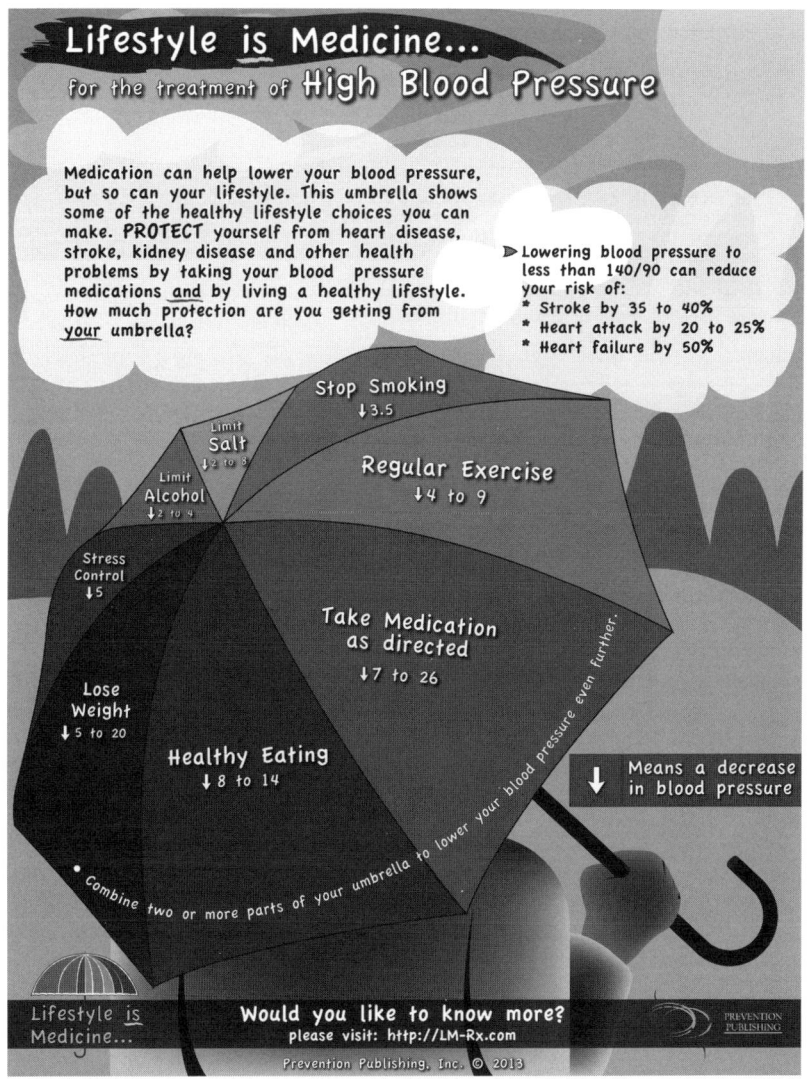

LM Tool H
Lifestyle is Medicine...for the treatment of High Cholesterol

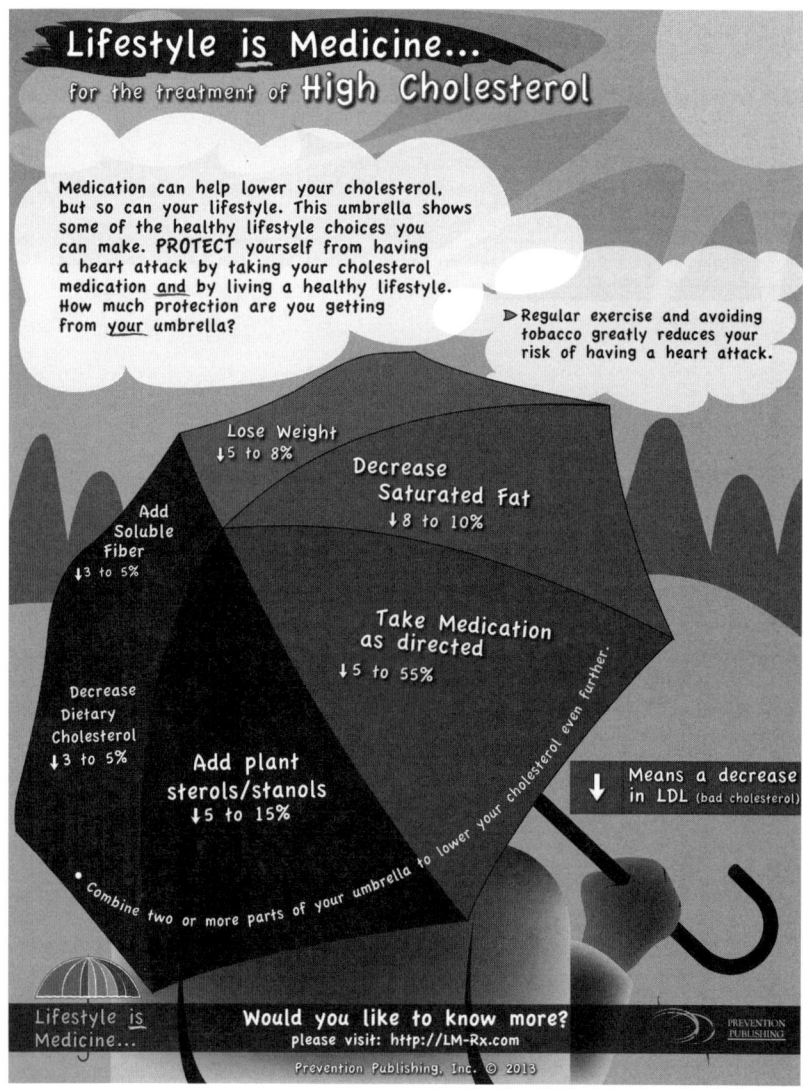

LM Tool I
Lifestyle is Medicine...for the treatment of Diabetes

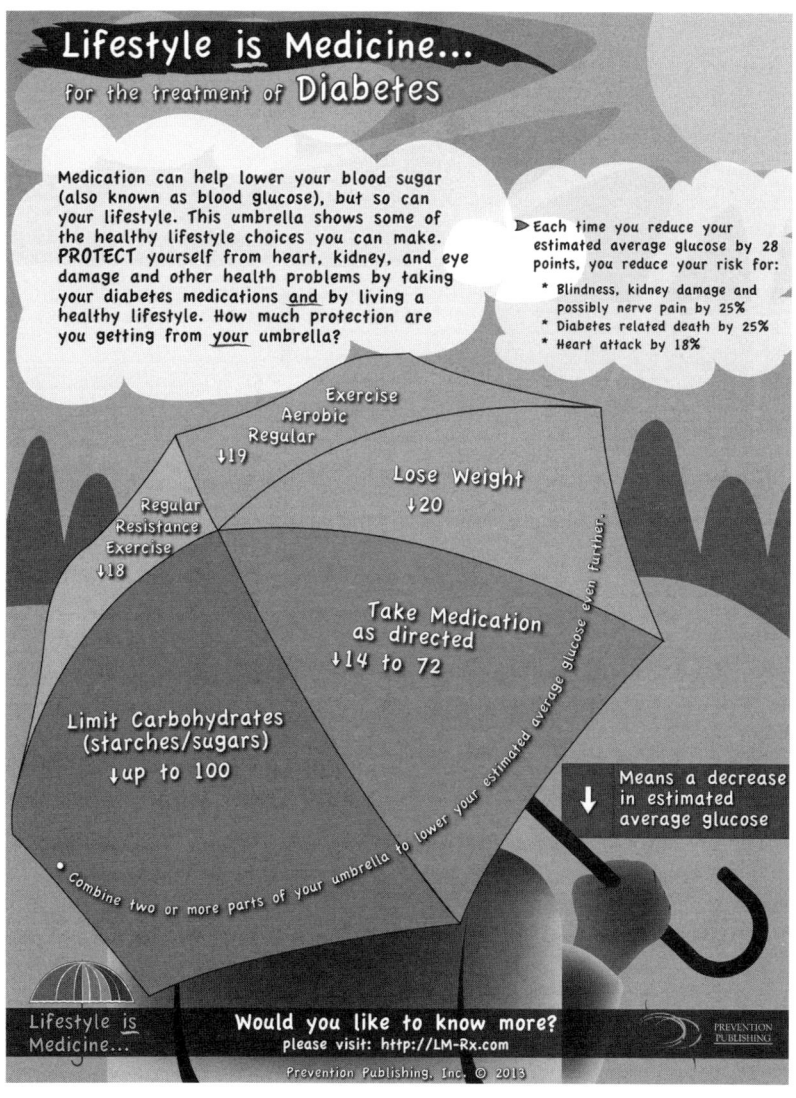

Test Your Knowledge - Answer Key

Chapter 1 1. c 2. a 3. d	Chapter 2 1. d 2. c 3. b	Chapter 3 1. b 2. d 3. b
Chapter 4 1. c 2. c 3. b	Chapter 5 1. e 2. c 3. b	Chapter 6 1. d 2. b 3. d
Chapter 7 1. a 2. b 3. c	Chapter 8 1. b 2. d 3. b	Chapter 9 1. d 2. d 3. c
Chapter 10 1. c 2. b 3. a	Chapter 11 1. c 2. c 3. b	Chapter 12 1. c 2. a 3. b
Chapter 13 1. a 2. d 3. a	Chapter 14 1. a 2. a 3. a	Chapter 15 1. a 2. a 3. b